The Qi Effect:

Chinese Energy Meets Quantum Biology to Enhance Your Personal Practice

by Francesco Garri Garripoli, D.D.

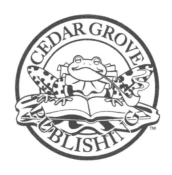

Table of Contents

Foreword

If I do make a stand in this book, it is that pretty much everything you have learned about Qi, the Chinese Taoist word for life-force energy - and energy in any cultural expression for that matter - has been wrong, really wrong. What we have "bought" as truth has kept both the Westerners who have embraced it, and the Chinese who revere it, in an unending loop of scarcity and limits. This paradigm of scarcity requires constant management for everything that we believe drains our life-force energy, and it comes with a built in reliance on others ranging from physicians and pharmaceuticals to big government. I have watched this paradigm of 'scarcity management' transform what was once a backwards country into the modern and powerful China of the 21st Century, yet at a dangerous price. Through this lens, it is easy to observe how these same developments are also unfolding in the United States, and throughout the entire Western world including India and Australia.

I argue that these growth changes are happening in an inefficient, inequitable, and dangerous way because of the gross misconception we hold about energy itself. Whether governments figure this out is a big question, but if we as individuals don't make the necessary shifts about life-force energy, sexual energy, and energy on every level, our health and our very freedom will be lost for the foreseeable future. Just as civil and voting rights activist Fannie Lou Hamer said back in the 1964, are you "sick of being sick and tired?" If you are, then it's time you work toward real and lasting solutions. Humanity has been dialed way back and it is time we change that.

This book is my attempt to offer a powerful and transformative solution. Together, we will explore the recent revelations in the fields of Quantum Biology and Epigenetics that have completely upended what we have thought about DNA and biochemistry. We will dive far into the realms of astrophysics and Black Holes to see how the latest findings about life-force energy on the cosmic scale are not what we've been led to believe. The entire journey of this book will bring us into the essence of the Qi Effect itself, to confirm that we are not the material bodies we thought we were and that how we look at energy needs to be transformed. We will see how, when interpreted correctly, ancient practices like Qigong fit perfectly into our evolution as a species on a body, mind, and spirit level.

When I first started reading about Eastern philosophies and higher consciousness back in the late 1960s, I secretly hoped that these esoteric subjects would enter the mainstream. I never imagined that 50 years later a "Qi charger" would recharge a smart phone or that terms like "energy medicine" would be casually dropped in everyday conversation. I was a young person searching intently for a like-minded community where I could discuss the nature of Mind, life-force energy, and explore all of my deep ontological questions. Since the internet had not yet been invented, I was mailing self-addressed, stamped envelopes to every "spiritual" and "alternative" organization I could find. I would anxiously wait weeks for the mailman to deliver me the replies in my the pre-stamped envelope I was required to send them. It didn't really match my vision of the fantasy where I, the willing adept, would meet the Master up on the mountaintop to absorb koan after koan of graciously imparted wisdom… but I took what I could get as a curious youngster… not many years later though, I would be meeting many Masters on many mountaintops…

Like many in the '60s and '70s, I looked to cultures other than my own Italian-American one for solutions, believing that Eastern philosophies held the answers to the questions of life that were plaguing the modern world.

In these current times, it's important to see how cultures, countries, and even individuals view energy of every kind. This may seem like a subtle point, and although this book focuses mainly on health, psychology, and a little spirituality, energy lies underneath it all. In a world where we are facing an "energy crisis," we have to see how fossil fuel energy, "green" energy, and bio-vitality energy are all deeply entwined. This perspective shift is critically necessary for all aspects of life from economy to healthcare. Just 50 years ago, Henry Kissinger, Nobel Prize winner and ex-Secretary of State, said in no uncertain terms, "Who controls energy can control whole continents; who controls money can control the world." If that globalist power-grab attitude doesn't scare you into claiming your own, sovereign energy, I don't know what will…

The fact is, if we don't learn to embrace and apply these emerging concepts about energy, we will most likely continue to be unhealthy and ultimately perish as a species on Earth. This book will show you how we've been duped into focusing on just surviving instead of fully thriving, and how we've been conditioned to constantly manage things rather than efficiently transforming them.

Who would have guessed that a Google search for the word "Qi" (pronounced "chee") would fetch 188,000,000 results in 0.49 seconds! "Prana" fetched only 49,400,000 results. I find the lower number of search results for Prana peculiar in light of the epic interest the public has taken in Yoga these days. Prana, a powerful and ancient word within the yogic tradition, means virtually the same thing as Qi. The significantly lower number of results for "Prana" might suggest that the majority of people practicing Yoga today are more concerned with fitness and stress-management than with the concept of life-force energy, and this reflects typical mainstream attitudes of materialism. Yet, "Qi" seems to remain curiously in vogue, perhaps especially so with the increasing rise of China on the world stage.

In the Chinese language, the ancient word for "Qi" is written in a beautiful calligraphic character that literally stands for "steam and rice." This suggests, in the traditional poetic and mystic Taoist fashion, the very practical yet esoteric nature of "life force energy." This character and its meaning originated in what is now China. Remember that that country was no more called "China" back in the days of Lao Tzu and the Taoists in 600 BCE than Italy was called "Italy" in the times of the Romans. We live with many misconceptions…

For thousands of years, people have been debating, questioning, refuting, exploring, lying, guessing, fantasizing, and experimenting all in the name of Qi. The ancient Hindus in India referred to this energy as Prana, while their contemporary Greeks named it Pneuma. In West African culture, you would use the word Ase, while Zulu wisdom uses Umoya. Hebrew culture refers to life energy as Ruah, while indigenous First Nations people of the Americas held it as Manitou. Hawaiians use the word Mana to describe this energy, Japanese know it as Ki, and Tibetans named it Lüng. The concept of "life-force energy" that in this book we will refer to as "Qi", has been part of nearly every culture throughout human history.

The following chapters will focus mainly on the Chinese perspective of Qi as I set out to challenge many of the ancient concepts that have been laid out in books and texts since the mythical Yellow Emperor started to outline Qi and its role in the healing arts. My intention is not to go about proving or disproving the existence of Qi or the many attributes people have attached to it. Nor do I make any attempt to establish and take a stand on any theory or principle. This book is a departure point of inquiry, an exploration that I have spent my life engaged in. Any theories or ideas presented in this book are done so in this spirit of exploration to gently encourage you to wander deeper into the nature of life-force energy from the "inside out." How can this journey to the Heart of life itself benefit you in your life? This is a personal, experiential journey for you to feel and put to the test these ideas in your body, mind, and spirit. Anything less would be a game of the ego and intellect. This life is not about believing all of the things you read in books. It's is about using what you read to stimulate your curiosity and nudge you to look inside yourself in order to know and feel what resonates deeply within your Heart resonant, Intuitive Mind… the aspect of your Mind that is neither intellectual nor survival based but rather connected and interwoven into the Quantum field itself.

In the last 25 years or so, Qigong has been seen more and more in mainstream awareness. Qigong is the practice of "working with Qi." The Chinese character for "Gong" refers to "work" or "discipline." Mainstream interest in Chinese concepts of Qi began with Bill Moyer's 1994 documentary on alternative healing that included a segment on Qigong, and continued with my own PBS-TV documentary "Qigong - Ancient Chinese Healing for the 21st Century" in 1998. Nielsen Ratings showed that my documentary was seen by 88 million PBS-TV viewers. This astounded everyone including PBS corporate, especially in those very early days of the internet. I remember funding the documentary myself because PBS didn't believe that anyone would want to watch an hour program talking about Chinese Qi, and they never paid me a penny for it. The fact is, it was in heavy rotation around the U.S., throughout Europe - and even in Canada thanks to my dear Daisy Lee. PBS-TV stations even began using the documentary for their own fundraising after they started receiving numerous calls to their local TV stations from viewers asking to find out when the documentary would air so they too could learn about Qi and Qigong.

When I made the documentary, I had been living in China for a number of years studying Eastern healing techniques that interested me enough to leave a full-ride scholarship in medical school at the University of Colorado. What I saw as limited, specialized, and increasingly pharmaceutically-based practice in Western allopathic medicine, was in fact person-centered and holistic in Traditional and Classical Chinese Medicine (TCM/CCM). Studying in China with various elder TCM, CCM, and Qigong Masters was fascinating, and led me to realize that I needed to create this television documentary (and write my first two books) to share my perspectives with the world. The best parts of Chinese culture inspired me, and gave me deep insights into the concept of Qi in terms of what bonded that country together, fed its spirit, and drove it to acquire wealth at such a rapid rate. In Mandarin, the word "China" is not used to refer to the country of China. Rather, it is called by the name "Zhong Guo." "Zhong Guo" translates to "Center Country." To feel you are the "country at the center of everything" carries a deep belief system within it. For me, understanding the concept of "Qi" helped me to understand why that was so. It can also help us to understand why China is developing at the rate and style it is, and how it has become a global power with massive influence in nearly every country around the world. The writing was on the wall when I was videotaping my documentary in the early-1990's. Now, those scenes I shot of hundreds of people riding bicycles and practicing Qigong in the park are but a distant memory in modern China just 30 years later…

With many of the Qigong Masters being well over 90 years-old at the time I was studying with them in China, I felt the urgency to complete my documentary. I knew they wouldn't be around for much longer, and I could see that China was rapidly changing before my eyes. One of these old wizards who lived in Beijing was Master Duan Zhi Liang. This amazing character we affectionately called Master Duan, was a Taoist. To add to his allure, he was also a devout Catholic. When I returned to the U.S. to complete the editing of the television documentary I met Daisy Lee and taught her the Qigong form I had learned from Master Duan. She and I soon brought the vibrant 94 year-old to Canada for his first time outside of China. Since he was prominently featured in the documentary, we visited several TV stations in Canada that Daisy had contacts with, along with stations in the U.S. that I had contacts with from when I won an Emmy Award for work I had done with PBS-TV years before. Everywhere we went with the spry old Master Duan he made a splash. It seemed that people needed to be convinced that this high-energy, senior Qigong doctor was actually real!

The bigger, underlying question people had was, "Is Qi energy and everything we've heard about it real as well?" You yourself may be wondering about the role of Qi in your life, and why you should even care about an ancient Chinese concept in these modern, high-tech times. What beliefs about Qi are already out there? Should we take them at face value just because they have been around in books for hundreds of years? What is "Qi Activation" and the "Qi Effect" anyway, and do these hold any validity within the scientific world? Is there a practical way to gain more energy and live a healthier life without depending on pharmaceuticals? Can we break our destructive habitual patterns and move from just surviving to truly thriving? Perhaps one or more of these questions have challenged you as they have for me over the past several decades. Read on and discover just how much we have been told about life-force energy that is wrong, really wrong. Breathe deep and enjoy the journey...

Everything They've Been Telling You About

Qi Energy Has Been Wrong

Each time a discussion begins about something theoretical or intangible, the legitimacy of the conversation is in dangerous territory. Speaking of the intangible requires each opinion and angle to rest upon speculations and theories that can never be completely and fully proven. If the intangible phenomena could be 100% accounted for, we would immediately emerge from the world of the theoretical into the realm of the verifiable.

"Qi" is the ancient Chinese Taoist concept of "life force energy", and is fundamentally theoretical because we can't measure it, let alone see it. Even so, literally millions of people around the world base their personal self-healthcare practice and professional healing treatments on it.

To be scientifically verifiable, the object in question must be measurable. Once the object is measured, the experiment needs to be replicated, measured and verified by others in a similarly scientific manner. This is the nature of modern science since the 16th Century CE. For the thousands of years that came before the scientific revolution and its standardized methods, the nature of "knowing something to be true" was simply what everyone believed to be true in accordance with the existing power structure. What you experienced or even felt to be true could easily be part of the belief system of your tribe, village, or country. Early Akkadian and Sumerian creation myths date back to 3,500 BCE. These myths, including one of my favorites, "The Epic of Gilgamesh," were in fact not myths at all to the people who lived by them. Rather, they were the unquestioned truths of nature, life, religion, and the energy behind accepted reality itself. No one questioned these creation stories because they composed the very fabric of their belief system and of existence itself. The Goddess Inanna could not been touched or seen except in the form of a statue, and was absolutely real. Her energy that created and destroyed life was palpable, and your very worship of her determined the outcome of your health. By the time cuneiform was developed and these "myths" were written down on clay tablets that remained preserved over the centuries, many of these beliefs were already ancient. Bits and pieces of them made their way into the Indian Vedic writings and even into the Old Testament Bible. The earliest recording of the idea of a universal creative force actually came from the writings of Zarathustra approximately 2,000 - 1,500 BCE - in ancient world near Mesopotamia in what is now Persia with the concept of "aša." Aša eventually became assimilated into the Hindu and Greek cultures, and has influenced everything from Buddhism to Western Philosophy.

Qi is life-force energy and cannot be touched or seen despite the claims of certain people who say they can feel it. As such, it can't be directly measured or observed. Even so, its effects and influences are fully accepted by millions around the world who can attest to what happens to them when they practice Qigong and begin to "feel" Qi in their bodies. The healing benefits of Qigong's mind-body interventions can be seen in "outcome research" conducted by well documented by researchers from high-caliber institutions such as Harvard University. Outcome research does just that, it documents specific outcomes of a decision. In this case, the positive outcome of practicing Qigong have been tracked in this research to increase heart rate variability and improve people's success in managing their stress, a leading cause for disease and illness. Other research outcomes from Stanford University show benefits in treating musculoskeletal disorders and cardiovascular disease. New studies are constantly being run, and show the efficacy of Qi-based healthcare practices.

Even with the top university researchers studying these healthcare benefits, direct measurement of Qi is impossible. Such is the dilemma of this wonderful, if not mystifying, exploration.

I have been the Chairman of the Qigong Institute, a wonderful and high-integrity non-profit organization devoted to research relating to Qigong and Energy Medicine, since its founder, Dr. Kenneth Sancier, passed me the torch in the mid-1990's. Dr. Sancier was a retired Senior Scientist at the Stanford Research Institute, a prestigious organization created the trustees of Stanford University, and a highly respected figure in the scientific community. For him to have interest in Qigong and write a seminar paper on the subject was a surprise to his peers. He helped bring credibility to what research had been going on in China for decades by merging it with Western science research protocol. Dr. Sancier has since passed, and I was honored to bring on Tom Rogers as the current President of the Qigong Institute. Tom, a dear friend and top Silicon Valley engineer, has taken the database of research that Dr. Sancier started and evolved it over the years to contain more than 17,000 entries with a massive amount of research from around the world, including top institutions like Harvard University, the National Institutes of Health's Complementary, and Alternative Medicine Department. As a volunteer like me, Tom has done a stellar job to help bring Qi into focus for those curious and wise enough to explore.

Qi, or "life force energy," as we will sometimes refer to it as, is a concept that is represented by a beautiful Chinese character which I will further describe later as it is quite fascinating. This character first appeared in ancient times and always carried a sense of mystery, relating to "rising vapors that form the clouds and all things.' It was later used in the early Taoist writings of the Tao Te Ching discovered in excavations from the late 4th Century BCE, though its authorship has been credited to the 6th Century BCE sage Lao Tzu, and carries esoteric references to the power of nature deep within us, all around us, and far into the Universe. The character appeared a few times in Confucian literature around 500 BCE, but was curiously attached to topics surrounding moral conduct and an individual's character which had nothing to do with what the rebellious and eccentric Taoists believed. The common Chinese character we now have for Qi was adopted in the early Han Dynasty around 210 BCE.

We can see that this powerful and deep concept was well established in ancient times. Concurrently in Greece, the concept of "Pneuma" was well established as the description of "life force energy." The ancient Hindu concept of "Prana" similarly describes the energy behind all of creation that keeps us alive and healthy. It's likely that the origin of this concept, which came through the writings of the Vedas written in an ancient language variant derived from Sumerian literature, can be traced back to the beginning of written history itself. Cultures that have thrived without ever having a written language, such as the Hawaiian culture, have no way of dating the origin of their own concepts of life force energy. The Hawaiian's word for life-force energy is "Mana." As such, humans have most likely explored the source of what sustains life in and around us since we became sentient. Understanding creation myths and how a culture views fundamental concepts about life gives you great insight into what drives them forward, what their strengths and weakness are, and how they relate to other cultures.

Like all concepts, Qi evolved over time. We can look at the etymological journey of a word to find its road map and trace its evolution as a concept throughout the ages. In Chinese, a single character is usually made up of two radicals: two elements that make up the complete character. One radical generally denotes the sound of the spoken word, while the other contains its essential meaning. Both create the whole. When I lived in China, I used my time between Qigong studies to practice calligraphy. The beautiful Chinese locals loved to help me, and I learned new characters every day. Practicing them over and over to get the feel of them, I realized there is a specific energy to the writing, more like painting, of Chinese characters: each character is a symbolic picture. This is completely different from the alphabetical constructions of words that point to a concept in the Western world. Research shows that the brain has a neurological response when a person looks at a painting or the calligraphy of a "flower" ('hua' in Mandarin) that is different from the neurological response the same person has reading the alphabetized word "f-l-o-w-e-r." We know that the brain's powerful neural synapses generate quantum energy fields, and that these coherent states give us access to reality as we know it.

The brilliant Ancient ones created a very powerful character to represent Qi. How in the world does one depict such a complex concept as "life force energy"? They took a written character "radical" that in 500 BCE had already been around for about a thousand years. This radical was originally used in sacred carvings used for tomb offerings. As the culture evolved, the radical's other-worldly, non-physical attributes carried over as it came to mean "air," steam, or gaseous ether. This radical was then combined with another radical, the one for uncooked rice, and together they became the Qi character we know today. How could these two unlikely elements for "steam" and "rice" combine to represent one of the most amazing concepts in human ontology?

When I was living in China in the early 90's, I asked 93 year-old Master Duan Zhi Liang, the elder with whom I studied acupuncture, bagua martial arts, tui na massage, and Qigong, about this curious Qi character. He laughed as he did when he began to prepare either for martial arts sparring or to explain advanced metaphysical concepts. In his determined and calculated way, h got out his calligraphy paintbrush and ink. On a large sheet of white paper he painted three parallel, horizontal lines. From the end of the third line, his brushstroke painted a nearly vertical downward line with a little hooked tail at the end. This he said was the sound "cheee" and that it represented "steam." I could see how its shape was related to "gaseousness"and "air" and so I nodded. He reminded me that steam is hot and therefore Yang in nature, formless, masculine, and "up on top," he added with his typical sardonic smile.

Beneath the three parallel lines he painted what looked like a "plus sign" and then added four more brush strokes from the center outwards to make it look like an "asterisk." He said that this was "meee" or rice: uncooked rice to be exact. Rice is cool, of the earth, and therefore Yin in nature. Solid and feminine, his eyes twinkled, emphasizing how it rests firmly underneath the Yang. I caught another sly smile from the Master.

Together, the masculine Yang "hot steam" and the feminine Yin "uncooked rice" form a dynamic process. On its own, neither element can fully represent "life force energy." Together though, they create cooked rice, an "edible food" that nourishes the human body. By itself, steam is scalding and can be dangerous. Uncooked rice is like tiny stones that can't be digested. It takes the dynamic alchemical merging of Yang and Yin to create something new, something useful, something more powerful than the sheer sum of its parts.

This "story" is actually a brilliant way to describe the complex process of Qi to everyday, ancient people. It's pretty good for us modern folks too because it moves away from the intellectual and esoteric "new age" languaging and brings us to the real essence of Qi. What could make more sense than to bring Qi "down-to-Earth" with the image of steam-and-rice? Life-force energy is what brings us sustenance and provides us with what we need to stay alive. Simple and to the point.

I believe that if we can't see Qi in this way, we will miss the point altogether and become lost in abstract, esoteric theory. This is the genius of the ancient Taoists in China. Make the complex simple, poetic, and approachable, and you've opened the door of curiosity to lure in those interested enough for further exploration. That is my intention here as well. As you read on, things will start to get more challenging, interesting, and hopefully a bit controversial.

According to a Taoist like Master Duan, Qi is not actually a fixed "thing" but more of a process - or maybe a driving force behind a dynamic process. It is the interplay between Yin and Yang, and within that dance Qi is activated. That said, Taoists still have a difficult time not describing Qi as a tangible thing. Talking about anything, even a concept, forces our intellectual minds to either give it physical characteristics or anthropomorphize it. To anthropomorphize is to project human-like qualities on something that is distinctly not human. It's what we do with our pets when we claim to understand their existence through our own frail human motives and emotions, the poor creatures.

It is our nature as humans to want to take this dynamic and extraordinary concept of Qi and apply curiously banal qualities to it, thinking that it can "flow" or become "stagnant," and even become "depleted" or "excessive." Over the millennia, Qi has at times been described to be "in excess." In other times, it has been considered "deficient." This very set of qualities has grown to become the foundation of what we know as Traditional Chinese Medicine (TCM) and as such, the bedrock principles for acupuncture, herbal medicine, tui na massage, Qigong exercise, and Qigong energy healing (classified as Medical Qigong). These concepts and qualities of Qi have been in place since the legendary Yellow Emperor Huang Di was first believed to have laid out what we know as TCM around 2,500 BCE. In fact, what was actually written in his name didn't appear in literature until the Warring States Period of China between 475 - 221 BCE. From what I have seen in many private museums during my travels across China over 25 odd years, it is clear that TCM evolved from a very primitive form with theories that fit the knowledge structure at the time. Modern times and morays have conformed TCM with Western Medicine so that they can coexist. In fact, TCM has been forced to fit into the insane allopathic healthcare system we see today in the U.S. and around the world, even in China. I remember seeing "Bian stones" in a Chinese medical university collection in the ancient capital of Xi'an. A sweet professor bribed a guard with a few sweet potatoes to let me inside the museum where only Chinese professors and State officials were allowed. True story, and the video footage I shot that day is in the documentary I produced and aired on PBS-TV back in 1998. These Bian stones were carbon dated to roughly 2,500 BCE, which put them around the time of the Yellow Emperor's supposed reign. They were used to affect the "flow" of Qi both through a type of "tui na" energy massage and acupressure. Since at that time the technology for manufacturing fine needles didn't exist, it was Bian stones, with their pointed ends, that were the precursor to acupuncture needles. Eventually in the Han Dynasty, around 200 BCE, metallurgy allowed the use of iron to make needles that created the beginnings of acupuncture. I did see many early needles in that museum from the Han Dynasty period, and I'll tell you that I'm not sure my Qi could have handled having these massive spikes piercing my skin. They looked more like railroad ties than the fine acupuncture needles in use today. It was good for a laugh from the professor when he saw my face. My sense was that people of ancient times may have gotten instantly cured seeing their doctor raise one of these massive needles, pleading that their Qi no longer needed treatment!

The point here is that in China, it took literally thousands of years to experiment and test theories around Qi and how to work with it in the human body. Why even "work" with Qi? Well, we are told that Qi flows through our bodies in "channels" called Jing Mai. In English we know these as meridians. We are also told that Qi flows around the outside of our body in an amorphous space called the "Wei Qi Field." It is believed to permeate the Universe, flowing out and around into space. We've been told that when Qi is blocked or stagnant, it leads to disease and illness that can manifest on a physical or emotional level. With all that we've heard about Qi, it makes sense to work with something that can improve our health, well-being, and even provide us with rejuvenation and longevity.

Since the Yellow Emperor's time, Chinese doctors, philosophers, and sages have all added their perspective to the concept of Qi. Papers have been written over the centuries, comments have made about the papers, and comments have been made about the comments. The Taoists have fabulous lineages of doctors, known as Dai Fu, who experimented with techniques ranging from breathing exercises to herbal formulas. You can look at lineage maps to see where a doctor experimented right up to the point that he died trying some formula or technique that didn't quite pan out… and then his or her protege picked up where they left off and continued experimenting. Taoists see themselves as part of the experiment: they were renowned for using their own bodies as laboratories to explore the limits of Qi and the human body. I have infinitely more respect for those courageous Taoists than I do for the physicians these days who prescribe Big Pharma medications that they would never themselves.

As knowledge amassed over time, it became clear not that Qi was "something" that needed to be managed, but that it had different "types." For example, "Jing Qi" is often referred to as Prenatal Qi. "Jing Qi" is believed to come from our ancestral line from our parents and their parents and so on. We receive it when we are born, and whatever amount we receive is all we will ever get. It's believed to reside mainly in the Kidney System region of our bodies and is slowly depleted as we age. Thus, Children have more Jing Qi than most adults. Luckily for us, there are ways to work with this Qi (remember, the art of Qigong means to "work with Qi" so this practice is key to embracing Qi) in order to retain as much as you can for as long as you can. There is a detailed Taoist science of sexual Qi-building and Qi retention. The idea is that we "deplete our Qi" through sexual release both in men and women, though more so in men. By reorienting the orgasm to retaining our semen or eggs, we can slow the depletion of Jing Qi. I will comment more on this later, and offer a reorientation that may surprise you.

Another type of Qi is simply referred to as "Qi" and is the life force energy that flows through the body on a day-to-day basis. It's what powers our metabolic system and our autonomic systems: blood circulation, digestion, breathing, and so on. It's what we rely on when we walk or run. It's the fuel, so to speak, that keeps us alive. It's believed that this Qi can be out of balance, depleted, or in excess. It is thought to even become stagnant and blocked. TCM techniques such as acupuncture, herbal medicine, and tui na massage all help to bring Qi into harmony, flow, and alignment. A wide variety of Qigong techniques focus on "collecting Qi" and storing it in the region of the Lower Dantian, in the abdomen below the navel. It's believed that gathering Qi and bringing it into the body will replenish your reserves. There are also ideas about "leaking Qi" where you lose Qi in various situations such as when you have an excessive emotional reaction, perform excessive exercise, or partake in excessive alcohol consumption. Oh yes, too much sex is also believed to deplete your Qi. Even exposure to the elements like wind and cold are considered "invasive" and are thought to affect your Qi.

The third "type" of Qi that is commonly taught based on ancient text is Shen Qi. We can think of this as "spirit" energy. Just as Jing is related to the past due to its ancestral, body-genetic associations, Shen is related to the future. This aspect of Qi propels us into the future, as its spirit-level energetic helps us unfold who we are at our essence in this moment to become what we shall become as we move ahead in life.

These concepts I'm sharing are just the first few that come to mind of the many I have studied, deeply considered, practiced, and taught to many thousands of students in workshops around the world over the last few decades. I believe there is a figurative and essential "truth" to each of these ideas. Many, many teachers in China and in other countries have impressed upon me the merits of these concepts, and I have been a good student by putting them to the test in my daily practice. I've studied and practiced acupuncture in China with great Master-level Dai Fu teachers to help many people, including my Mom who couldn't find pain relief in the world of allopathic medicine she so trusted. I've studied tui na massage for some 20 years from great, Master-level instructors. I've studied Qigong with many great elder Masters in China and around the world, learning everything I could of this wonderful healing art that combines breathing techniques, specific movements, and postures with mental focus and visualization. All this has benefitted me, clients, and the students who have studied with me greatly, yet I have discovered through dedicated practice that by making subtle changes in how I engaged with Qi, amazing results were possible.

The following chapters will share what I have come to and what has taken people's personal practice to the next level.

Much to the chagrin of my dear parents, I left a full-ride medical school scholarship at the University of Colorado, Boulder back in the mid-70s so that I could head toward Asia to study Eastern healing with an 81 year-old Master. I knew then at 18 years old that there was more to true, holistic healing than the Western allopathic medical model could offer me. I had spent hours in private discussion after my pre-med classes talking with my professors, asking them questions about holistic healing. I wanted to understand the role of the mind and energy in the way the body heals. Remember that in the mid-1970s this was not the normal conversation at a big university, but it was Boulder after all and that little mountain college town was one of the epicenters of consciousness exploration. Each professor told me the same thing: becoming a Western physician would never serve my spirit or answer my questions. The allopathic model had no contextual framework for what I was interested in pursing. I am infinitely grateful to those professors who took the time to sit with me in their homes off campus to meet me where I was, and to support my searching spirit. The answer seemed to be in Eastern Medicine and its philosophical, whole-person-healing model. A model that centered around the presence of Prana, Mana, and… Qi.

I was a good student and stayed with the Master teachers until the time came when they told me I was ready to go out and teach. With these old Masters it wasn't about "passing a test" and getting a certificate, it was about enduring their sometimes challenging, non-linear teaching process for long enough and with enough sincerity that they trusted you. This kind of "study" involved sleeping on clinic floors and waking up before sunrise to practice with the Master. It involved going into poor villages with the Master and providing 50-100 acupuncture treatments each day to every villager who chose to come and share their medical condition. I remember one time when I was taken to a village in the Chinese countryside that was so remote it involved passing through three military checkpoints. People forget that getting around inside China, even for the Chinese, is not an easy matter. The Master would have the driver of our beat-up pick-up truck pull over on the side of the road a few kilometers before each check-point and make me climb into the back of the truck. He and the driver would then cover me in cardboard and hay and tell me to stay quiet. I would hear the truck start back up and drive… and then we'd pull to a stop. I'd hear some conversation ensue in Mandarin that sounded very serious. The main word I would hear the Qigong Master say was, "Mei you" which means "We don't have." I presumed the fuller sentence to go something like, "No, we don't have any Italian-American Qigong student we are smuggling in the back of the truck under the cardboard and hay."

At the time, I thought it was all very exciting stuff to pass through checkpoint after checkpoint never being found out. I look back on those days now and wonder what would have happened if they had checked and found me. It did so happen that I was in fact arrested once during my travels in China, but I'll leave that for another book.

Studying with these Masters also involved participating in Qigong energy healing sessions that went on late into the night with dozens of elder Japanese cancer patients who came to Beijing in hopes of being healed by the Master and his students. Sometimes my studies required running at full speed up the Song Mountains behind the Shaolin Temple in the pre-dawn dark with a dozen young monks. Our upward sprint was but a preparation for the full day of training awaiting us back down at the temple with the elder Buddhist Master. We would sit and listen with earnest focus to hear what he had to say that day. This style of training involved fostering the patience to wait for when the "gems" of true insight and knowledge would be given by the Master. It anything but straightforward, and required going on errands with them, hiking deep into the mountain forests for days on end with them, and eating meals together. We went horse backing riding in the Mongolian steppes together and I drank their terrible "bai jiu" liquor with them, listening to their endless stories into the wee hours. Sometimes the stories repeated over and over. I became practiced at acting like every time was the first time I had heard that story. Then, unexpectedly, the "gem" of wisdom would emerge: a discourse on the nature of Qi, a method for improving digestion, a breath technique that, well, leaves you breathless. This is what studying with these senior Masters was like, and absolutely nothing about it remotely resembled my time at the university, thank heavens.

There is an ancient Taoist phrase that I have been sharing for decades to describe the relationship between Qi and the mind. Taoists referred to this as "Yi," the part of the conscious mind that sets intentions and visualizes concepts, objects, people, and so on. The literal translation of Yi is "Bringing Qi to Mind," and is a fabulous concept. These days, Yi is generally considered to mean "thinking" or "what you think." These interpretations are lacking, and the concept is largely misunderstood. The ancient intention within the concept of Yi is carried through the etymology of this character, referring to how we "activate" Qi through our conscious awareness. This is big, and is why Yi is one of the three key aspects of Qigong along with breathing techniques and movements/postures.

The ancient Chinese character "Tao" (Dao) to refer to "movement or guiding." It is sometimes thought of as "the way, the path," and is used in the ancient book, the Tao Te Ching, attributed to Lao Tze, the 6th Century BCE Taoist Master. The phrase is as follows:

"Yi Tao, Qi Tao."

Simple and beautiful, and as wonderfully complex, poetic, and rich as only Taoism can awaken in the human spirit.

You know the concept behind each character now, and so together we may translate this phrase as:

"Where the Mind goes, Qi goes."

This is a good starting point, although is the most basic interpretation of this powerful phrase. If we choose to leave this translation as is, we will become trapped in a limitation that so many who practice Qigong or the Qi-healing arts are in. As you read on, you will come to see a much different translation that reflects a deeper, more empowering view of Qi. The interpretation I will offer you departs from both the ancient tradition and what most modern practitioners and teachers hold to be true. With an open Heart-Mind, you will come to discover, as I have, that Qi doesn't "go" anywhere, but it is in fact activated.

In my early studies and practice in the art of "working with Qi" through the healing arts practice we call Qigong, I took the aforementioned phrase literally, just as my Master teachers had taught it to me. The idea was that wherever you "set" your "Yi", the Qi will move with it. In other words, if I set my intention to "bring" or "guide" Qi to an area of my body, the Qi will move and flow to that spot in some fluid-like way. Like so many Qigong and Tai Chi practitioners, I worked to direct Qi using my mind. All of my practice and meditation centered around this procedure in one way or another. Now, with many decades of practicing and listening to my Intuitive Mind guidance, I have come to understand the ways of Yi and Qi to be very different from the literal interpretations.

Ever since I was a young teen, I recognized the power of "mind." I constantly studied techniques to help me focus and develop the energy of my mind. These practices included various meditation techniques from all over the world including India, ancient Rome, and China, as well as various Western "mind enhancement" exercises coming from instructors in California. In the late '60's and early '70's, there were a plethora of organizations offering correspondence courses and booklets to be had for the asking. Suffice it to say, I spent a lot of the money I made on my paper route on payments for the courses, including a self-addressed, stamped envelope as was required in those days. My Dad became so frustrated that I was getting more mail delivered by the postman at 9 and 10 years old than he was.

I even used whatever technology I could get my hands on to explore the potential energy of my mind. As you may know, in the early-1970's one could don an analog electronic on their head to supposedly tap the latent ability of the brain. The device used flashing lights or sequential sounds to stimulate these latent, cranial recesses. Of course my parents and friends thought I was a bit eccentric wearing headsets bought from experimental labs purporting quasi-science. Since this was before affordable digital computer technology, these contraptions were largely hand-wired analog circuitry with minimal control knobs. To go further, I bought a soldering gun and rewired some of the circuit boards myself. I even designed my own devices in hopes of contributing to the new frontiers of this exploration. One day, I remember my poor Mom walking into my bedroom laboratory while I was mid-experiment. I had glued an array of mirror onto a piece of latex rubber, and had stretched the latex over a speaker. The music that played on the speaker was coming from an audio circuit I designed to synthesized frequencies I felt would positively entrain the brain to whatever intention I set. A light from a makeshift laser shot around the room, dancing across the mirrors that vibrated in sync with the audio frequencies. It must have looked and sounded like some strange, psychedelic gathering in Haight Ashbury. I sat in full-lotus amidst this freak-show. All my Mom could eek out before bursting into tears was, "Dinner is ready."

For someone like my beautiful Mom who was simply grateful for a mind that could successfully get her through the rigors of daily life raising 7 children, taking the effort or even seeing the need to enhance an already overworked mind was out of the question. For me and for many of us, we know intuitively that we have barely begun to tap the wealth of our mind. Knowing that humans only use 10% of our brain on average, I have remained inspired to keep pushing the envelope to discover the mysteries of our thinking process that remain hidden within that wondrous other 90%.

When I was taught that my mind could "guide Qi," I was obviously enthralled. I became a dedicated practitioner. A type of Qigong called "Nei Gong" focuses more on an inward level of the practice similar to guided visualization. My first entry into Qigong was through Nei Gong practice, as the Master teacher I studied with at the time didn't want me to focus my 18 year-old body in a physical way like most teenagers naturally do. This 81 year-old teacher had me focus on my "energy body" instead. Amongst his Eastern studies, he had personally studied with Carl Jung for years when he was a young man, and so he had a deep sense of the influence of the collective unconscious archetypes upon us.

It was this Master teacher's emphasis that always stuck with me. By not being allowed to focus on or be distracted by the physical, I was able to go on an inner exploration of life force energy. I learned that our true power is in our sensitivity, not force. At the core, Qigong for me is "sensitivity training." Qigong is about cultivating a sensitivity to Qi itself. By taking that deep-dive to look inside myself, I began to peer into the core of my true identity. This identity was not one based on my physical qualities, gender, age, race, or even the beliefs I had about myself. My "true" and authentic identity was one based on energy essence, defined in every way by Qi. Learning to tap into this infinite field of energetic resource on a body, mind, and spirit level is the only way that we can truly know who and what we are. In doing so, we become sovereign, whole, and complete as we accept our own perfection. This is a big shift from what I was told I was through my societal conditioning, and its a big shift from the "scarcity model" of the world that most everyone around me was ruled by.

We've all grown up with the concept that energy, along with most of life's resources for that matter, are finite. We've been told these resources are in a limited supply, a challenge to secure, and something that needs to be protected. Especially for the generation that came before me, experiencing two World Wars with the Great Depression in between, not to mention the oppressive ways of Communism, it is no surprise that a world view based on scarcity has come to dominate the global belief system. When resources like food, fuel, and money are limited, we begin to see our life force energy, whether you know about Qi or not, as something that is also limited. Our vitality, or "élan vital" as it is sometimes referred to in the West, is based on our world view. If that viewpoint is dominated by limits and scarcity, so is our vitality. Our education system, religious training, and government have all held these beliefs of energy scarcity to be the absolute foundation of decision making, commerce, international relations, and strategic planning. Most of the time, there were no bad intentions from these influencing systems: they simply evolved to protect and support us in the only way they knew how to in a world of limits and scarcity. When the systems that influence and control our everyday life are impressing ideas upon us of fear-based scarcity and limitation, it is difficult not to find ourselves buying into that belief system and running our daily lives accordingly.

It's important to see how we've been influenced, conditioned, and programmed to think the way we do. The way we think and what we believe to be true influences every aspect of our lives, from our choices on how to act and what to eat, to who we spend time with and what we actually think about. I'll dive deeper into these ideas later on by exploring the emerging science of Epigenetics and my concept of "Epimemes," but for now it's important to simply see how our conditioning has affected the very way we look at Qi and energy itself.

When we can begin to see that this conditioning is deeply based on Fear, then we can see how beliefs of scarcity and limits emerge directly from that Fear. The path of Truth, the "spiritual path" if you will, has always been one of courage, rising us up out of the grasp of Fear's darkness and into the light of the Heart. The word "courage" after all comes from the Latin root "cor" which means Heart.

If you are interested in pursuing this path of the Heart and transcending the limits of Qi that have been imposed on you, then the only recourse is to trust your Heart-centered intuition and take the courageous steps to learn another way of being. As I mentioned earlier, our Heart-resonant Intuitive Mind is that aspect of our Mind that is not bound by the linear intellectual bandwidth that measure and judges, nor is it the aspect of Mind that is consumed with survival-oriented processing. Our Heart resonance is that part of us - which the ancient Taoists referred to as Shen Qi - that opens us to our spirit, to that knowing that we are more than simply a physical, material entity. Feeling this is why you're reading this book and why you have been exploring new ways of thinking to shift the many aspects of your life you would like to change. Our lives are wrought with challenges stemming from energetic issues in our families, jobs, relationships, and health. You know what you are facing right now. It may be a major life issue. It might be just a subtle piece of the puzzle floating around, looking for its place in the whole picture of your life. It doesn't matter what it is, what matters is that this is what makes us human and transcending our limiting, materialistic beliefs sets us free.

It's time to explore the Qi Effect and see how this concept resonates with you. It may confront ideas and beliefs you've come to hold true. That is to be expected. Every explorer must push beyond the horizon, beyond all definitions of the known, comfortable, and familiar. Only in the beyond will you find the land of possibilities, amazing new resources, and worlds unknown that will change your reality forever.

The Origin of Everything

Ever since I was a child, I've been fascinated by the many different stories that explain how our Universe came into being. Maybe you were like that too. Maybe you were curious about the science, fascinated by the story of the Big Bang theory and the ever-expanding, infinite nature of it all. When I was young I didn't have a lot of friends who were interested in discussing these ideas. I noticed most kids typically wavered their interest between sports, eating, and socializing. I came to understand that that's what normal human kids do and what normal human parents seem to agree is worthwhile and important.

I remember how one day in fifth grade art class, the teacher bravely introduced our class to sculpting with clay. At one point, after several days deep into the project, I looked up at the room to see what the other students were making. Amongst the plethora of basic blobs and deformed animals there was the random bowl or plate. A few art classes later we proudly lined our creations on trays and prepared them for the kiln. I noticed all of the kids were staring curiously at my creation. It was my best attempt at Rodin's "The Thinker." You know, the man sitting on the stone with his elbow on his knee, chin perched on his fist. It was the image that came to me first at the thought of trying my hand at sculpture because it's an image I could relate to. This is how my Mind has always worked... full of endless curiosity and fearless questioning. In grade school, only the blessed librarians knew how to deal with me. They let me cut class and sit in a corner. I quietly weeded through the Dewey Decimal System, absorbing everything I could on science, ancient history, spirituality, and shamanic practices. I always had access to these books because they were never checked out and always on the shelf. What pressed me forward was my constant desire to grasp the energy that brought the known Universe into existence. I had the same questions that plagued every thinker: How did we get here? Was all we see really created in a flash? What, if any, is God's role in creation? What is the origin of life and consciousness?

Curiously, I didn't even think to ask anyone about these "creation questions" until I was 8 or 9 years old. Why? Before that I was completely at peace with feeling I already knew, and I naturally figured that others did too. I had such a strong feeling of knowing because all of my dreams at night were the same. I got into bed, closed my eyes as I fell fast asleep. During that "sleep" time, I entered "the dream." It was always the same and it was really quite simple. The dream's point-of-view was me staring into a star-filled sky. A proscenium, like the frame around a stage in a theatre, bordered the edges of the scene with back-lit clouds. These clouds were big, puffy cumulous clouds lit by something bright and out of view. I assumed it was the Moon or the stars themselves casting their light on the clouds. It was soft and beautiful. The whole of the dream was this picture of me staring peacefully at the stars. The star gazing lasted all night. There was no movement or activity, just a sense of being "at home" in this infinite starfield.

One day, I asked my Mom about these star field dreams we all have at night and if she enjoyed them as much as I did. She looked at me in that quizzical way and squinted her eyes. She said something like, "That sounds like you again, but it's not what your mother dreams about." Being an inquisitive little guy, I asked her about her dreams and she just shook her head and smiled. I began randomly asking adults about their starfield dreams and what it was like for them. I was met with the kind of faces people make when you tell them you think an alien is sitting on their shoulder. Some people would smile and say I was cute before changing the subject. Others laughed and offer me food, probably thinking that hunger had gotten the best of me. I did grow up in a big Italian community. This sort of feedback really had me convinced that these people did have starfield dreams and just thought I wasn't old enough yet to discuss them. I didn't give up continuing to randomly inquire. I started asking the kids at school and even asked around with my older teen cousins, but I always received the same response. I went from the insecure feeling that people were keeping a big secret from me to the conclusion, a tough one to accept, that adults really have no idea about anything deep or meaningful and that kids are simply adults-in-training.

I finally asked my question about starfield dreams to my Uncle Mike. He was one of those non-bloodline uncles that are everywhere in extended Italian families. Uncle Mike had a deep, sad soul and I figured that he might think about these types of things. If nothing else, he always brought me a toy when he stopped by, so he was definitely one of the "good guys." I'll never forget the day I took him to the side to ask him my big question. I was quite pleased that he'd just given me a Flexible Flyer sled, the ultimate gift an 8 year-old could ever receive. Once we were away from the rest of the chaotic family conversation, I asked him about his starfield dreams. Being the sensitive soul he was, he gently stared into my eyes and waited until I was finished. He took my hand and said without breaking eye-contact, "You are going to find out that everyone isn't exactly like you, and that most people don't see things the way you do or even ask the questions you do. Some things are best to keep to yourself." I took this as more of a global comment and not specifically about me and my dreams, so I didn't take it as personally as I should have. It also left me feeling that even Uncle Mike wasn't going to be any real help on the starfield dream issue, or on the whole "origin of life" question that I faced on the daily.

I remember finally settling in to the idea that I didn't need validation. My nighttime sojourns didn't need to be real, common, or really anything to other people. They were mine. When I gazed into the starfield, the sense that this was where we all came from permeated me. It was always there, without beginning or end: it just was and always was. Once I finally accepted that, the dreams stopped rarely ever to return.

The pace of scientific research picked up in the 1960s and ended the decade with the Apollo missions to the Moon. As technology advanced, theories about our origin continued to pour in. I always felt that the more intellectual studies a person pursued, the more indoctrinated they got into group-think, mainstream theories. I could see how intellectualization develops patterns of pigeon-holes and belief systems that disable free-thinkers from being able to trust their intuition. I watched as intellects bowed their heads to the research labs and publications. Then there was Edwin Hubble, whose work on doppler red shift revved up everyone who'd been waiting for the nail to finally drive the Big Bang Theory into a permanent place on the pedestal of truth. It's funny how people, especially scientists, can slide in mathematical equations to support their own viewpoint. The Hubble Constant gave the Big Bang proponents just what they needed to "prove" they were right. Science loves adding "constants" into mathematical equations, because assigning a constant value to a variable clears up a lot of messy things that otherwise can't be explained. The fact is, Hubble's theory doesn't work for objects in space that are farther than a billion light years away. Even though a billion light years away sounds like a really far away place, there are many, many objects that far and farther away. Anyone who desperately clings on to the Big Bang Theory will huff and dismiss you. They'll come up with yet another way to explain how one day 13.8 billion years ago, the whole universe spontaneously emerged out of a highly compressed point and suddenly exploded onto the scene to make everything you see around you today. Every time I even consider that people still actually believe this, I project into the future when this theory will be tossed into the same waste bucket that holds other throw away theories like "we live in an Earth-centered solar system" and "the Earth is flat."

In the last chapter, we discussed anthropomorphizing and the way humans project their own emotions and issues onto their poor pets. We humans have a tendency not only to project our issues and emotions, but our "human limits and traits" onto everything around us. While this brings certain people comfort, it drives me a little mad. People feel that if they were born, then the Universe itself must have been born too.

To continue my point about the group-think that runs the scientific world, I want to cover a recently discovered galaxy. This galaxy was poetically found by the Hubble Space Telescope. Yes, the telescope was named Hubble after the man who's constant allows us to use our Big Bang Birthday to determine both the finite size and age of our Universe. It is largely agreed throughout the whole of the global scientific community that the age of this new galaxy, named GN-z11 and located in the constellation of Ursa Major, is 13.4 billion years-old and is over 32 billion light years away. Do these numbers bother you like they do me?

How in the world could the Big Bang have occurred 13.8 billion years ago, and then just 400 million years later a complete and massive galaxy pops into existence at a distance more than double the supposed age of the Universe? The youngest galaxies that we are aware of are all at least 500 million years old and certainly not 32 billion light years away from ground zero. These numbers just don't add up.

So now you're brain hurts and you're asking why any of this is important in the first place. It's important because if the speed of light is the speed limit for matter in the Universe, how did GN-z11 get 32 billion light years away from the theoretical point of The Bang if the Universe isn't even that old? You then have to create a theory about how the Universe is expanding super-fast to make up the difference. What a fragile web we weave when we cling to concepts that fall apart right in front of us. When you read statements like the following from a respected PhD at UCLA, you can see that the game is to simply spew the accepted narrative in order to continue securing grant money. "We know the Universe went through a hot dense phase because of the light element abundances and the properties of the cosmic microwave background. These require that the Universe was at least a billion times smaller in the past than it is now." This statement exemplifies what is know as "closed loop logic." Saying that something is so because it references something you just said just doesn't make sense nor does it prove anything.

The point here is: don't believe anything at face value and you will begin to free yourself of the conditioning that has been limiting you in ways you've never even realized. Carl Sagan, an outspoken astronomer and scientist who influenced many during my youth, spoke years later, just before his passing in 1996, on how we must be skeptical of science, allowing all voices and views to be heard equally, rather than simply accepting the narrative of a government or a charlatan. He made it clear that science defines the cultural belief system of a society, so science must constantly be questioned and pushed to evidence-based testing.

There are fabulous debates trying to explain all of the current scientific theories and not one of them is convincing to me. Yet throughout history, facts rarely need to get in the way of a good and widely accepted mainstream theory. Ask poor Galileo. He was put under house arrest by the Church-influenced government for proving that the Earth was in fact not the center of our solar system. All that was required for him to make his point was a telescope along with years of data collection. Maybe it wasn't just that his findings were scientifically provable fact that concerned both establishments of church and science. Maybe instead, the deeper significance was that anyone with a telescope could pioneer the exploration of the universe on their own, and that was too threatening to the established narrative. Maybe it was that with just a little bit of free and intelligent thought, anyone could start finding holes within the existing canon of thought. Galileo's arrest may have had more to do with inspiring others to become free thinkers and explore on their own than anything else.

We have accepted that the images taken from the Hubble Space Telescope and NASA are "views of our Universe." If we sat by the window and looked out as we traveled the Universe by spacecraft, we would see something completely different. I know this sounds strange, but most of the color and detail in these "space" images are computer generated composites of visible light combined with "invisible light." Examples of what we call invisible light are x-rays, infrared, and radio waves. The human eye and optical brainwave processing do not perceive this light and register only a minute sliver of the available frequencies. We are literally blind to much of what exists in the world we live in, existing with massive perceptual limits. Technology can help us to "see" much more than we can with our native human vision, but technology is still only an extension of what we know. Technology simply amplifying or expanding upon that which is known, it does not show us what is not yet known. The Universe is comprised of so much that we don't yet know, and we haven't yet designed technology to assist us in "seeing" into the unknown. The tiny percentage of what we see with our natural and even tech-supported senses is but a mere fraction of what actually exists in this Universe. To accept that will help us to prepare us for true discovery.

As I now share a slightly different view of cosmology, I trust you will bring an open mind. As we can see, the "best minds" in science can't fully agree on the big picture. They lack solid proof of their Big Bang origin-story and are having a difficult time maintaining it as more and more new information is uncovered. The 1965 discovery of "cosmic microwave background" seemed to be a winner of convenient explanations for some, though not all, of the the Big Bang theory. The "cosmic microwave background" is believed to be the thermal remnant left over from the Big Bang moment, and the oldest light that exists. Since 1896, measurements have been made to calculate this microwave temperature in outer space. As technology improves the temperature we measure changes along with their corresponding theories, the supposed "proof" of the Big Bang. I counted nearly 100 changes in these explanations since 1896. To this very day as discoveries are made that continue to chip away at the theory, science comes up with another way to explain the anomalies away and continue clinging to the Big Bang. Mainstream science even had to come up with the concept of "inflation" and create stories of the "first second after the Big Bang" in order to account for the smoothness of mass distribution in the Universe that they couldn't explain. In the 1980's, the mainstream added in explanations for new anomalies and came up with theories like dark matter and dark energy. They are still struggling to keep their story straight.

Astronomers and astrophysicists now believe that the universe is expanding, through what they call "cosmic inflation." This belief stems from their Big Bang theory and it supports what I feel is an illusory misinterpretation of the truth. Cosmic inflation is an observational convenience to explain away the Doppler shift they see in space telescopes. This describes why stars have a red-shift in their spectrum, which in basic physics indicates that an object is moving away from you. To the traditional physicists, this can only mean that all the stars in the universe are moving away from us at increasing speed over time. Curiously, this is also occurring at equally distributed vectors radiating from our point of view on Earth in every direction. In other words, this observation puts us at the very center of this expanding universe. Convenient, but not likely.

To me, this is akin to when the scientific community (and the religious leaders at the time) believed that the Sun and planets revolved around the Earth. When poor Galileo showed through rigorous observation that it was actually the Sun that was at the center of all planet orbits, remember that he was placed under house arrest. People don't easily accept challenges to their belief system, especially if it threatens the whole of their narrative.

Think how ancient sailors were convinced that the Earth was flat as they looked outward, believing the oceans extended only as far as the edge of the flatness before falling off. Scared to sail too far away, their fear spawned myriad stories of sea monsters and explorers who "fell off the edge." Like those who believed that the Earth was the center of planetary and even solar orbits, the flat Earth world view came from the natural, if erroneous, tendency to feel that you are at the most important location in the universe: at the very center of it all. Remember that the ancient Chinese named their country "Zhong Guo," meaning "center country," believing that they were the very center of the world.

I have come to realize that this same tendency has influenced even modern astrophysicists. The propensity to be so material-based and Earth-centered has confused many scientific views, including the cosmic inflation theory. It is not that the stars and galaxies are moving away from us in every direction, but it is actually that WE are moving away from them. How could that be? We are simply experiencing a space/time contraction in our local galactic starfield as it steadily collapses into Sagittarius A*, our local black hole at the very center of the Milky Way. That would easily explain what we are experiencing in this illusion of an "expanding universal space/time." It's actually just the opposite of current scientific thinking even though it creates the same observational illusion.

If the universe is in fact expanding as science believes, then how do we explain the prediction that our nearest galactic neighbor, the Andromeda galaxy, will engulf the Milky Way in 4.5 billion years? How can this local gravitational compression effect explain away the expansion that astrophysicists are trying to sell us?

If what we are experiencing is instead the space/time collapse that Einstein's general relativity theory explains occurs around super-massive black holes, then it would make sense to think that everything in the universe from OUR point of view is moving away from us at a relatively equal rate in every direction. I imagine it may actually turn out that we are slowly falling into the event horizon of the super-massive Sagittarius A*, a slow and steady descent into this black hole 4 million times the mass of our Sun. Granted, Sagittarius A* is 26,673 light years from us, so you may question any effect on Earth if its core event horizon is believed to be only 37 million miles in size. This super-massive black hole is strong enough to hold all ~400 billion stars in the Milky Way galaxy in its gravitational field, which is 185,000 light years across. We are a spiral galaxy because this black hole holds all these stars in their orbits around it, including our Sun. That is just from the force of gravity, which we know is one of the weakest forces measured. We really have no idea of what subtle space/time warping occurs at large distances since most observations are of easy to observe things like gravitational lensing or accretion rings around black holes.

How curiously does this also mirror what is taking place on Earth with large financial systems, governments, and corporations expanding in size like never before in history and drawing everything into their grasp? If we allow this trend to occur, we will see our freedom moving away from us at the same speed stars and galaxies appear to be escaping from our current point of view.

When I was a kid we had to say answer that "Saturn has 8 moons" in order to pass the science test. That answer was simply the truth back then. Nowadays, the right answer is 82. Yes, 82. Science can only explain what the senses can detect in that moment. Moments pass and moments change, so we know that very soon the story will change, again. If we stay locked on this roller coaster of our limited senses, we will forever be on an endless ride. When we can finally disengage from the need for "scientific truth," we will free our Intuitive Mind to see beyond the shackles of our five senses and truly be liberated.

There are a myriad of "origin" stories from our ancient predecessors. Most are poetic and fabulous, involving god-like beings that live together on mountaintops or emerge from the stars. We must remember that each of these stories arose from the contextual framework of the culture at the time. Most of these origin stories came at a time when there was a tribal leader such as a king, queen, or pharaoh. As a result, oftentimes the "original creator" appeared similar to, or "similar to and a bit better than," the leader in power. Amongst all of the different fantastical explanations for the story of our world, there was a common consensus that the creation of this amazing place was an appropriately amazing act. Such an act of creation could only be accomplished by an equally amazing being who created something from nothing. In some stories, it took nothing more than a spoken word. Although the stories varied, it was clear that the whoever had done the creating was a great creator who had existed beforehand. Nobody knows exactly what they sat on or where they slept before they did the creating, that mysterious world of the before was simply an unimportant albeit mystifying detail.

It's easy to see that science and materialism have gained dominance as humanity steadily moves away from being spiritually-oriented and toward an intellectually-oriented world view. The 500 years since the Newtonian revolution of empirical physics and material science have brought a near-total push for a physical explanation of everything and a celebration of all things intellectual. This recent, half-millennium phase in human history has moved us away from a spiritually-based, energy-oriented, right-brain, intuitive matriarchal world-view, and into a materialistic, left-brain, intellectually patriarchal world-view. There are many, many examples of this. Since evolution is a slow and subtle process, it's incredibly difficult to notice the shifts happening all around us. Ask any frog placed in a pot of cool water to narrate his environmental changes as the flame turns up and the waters start to heat. The frog barely notices that something has changed before he becomes part of the boiling soup. We're not much different than frogs from time to time…

So it's no doubt that the Big Bang Theory appears as a seductive solution for the creation of everything. The cultural shift away from spiritual beliefs into hard material science has required that we eliminate the "creator" persona from our currently held origin story. We rationalized away an almighty creator, but we couldn't get rid of the "creation" process itself. It's easy enough for the scientifically oriented mind to eliminate the possibility of "the creator," but the mapping and conditioning of the creation-story is too deep to eliminate. Science may be seductive and the mathematics may be elegant, but the conclusions are flawed… and more and more clear-thinking physicists and mathematicians are starting to question everything we have believed to be true about the world we see around us.

This book is called "The Qi Effect" because the point of our exploration together is to grasp the absolutely energetic nature of our apparent "physical" reality. Let's begin by going on a journey to see an alternative explanation for how the Universe came into being. Let's hear an origin story that from an energetic perspective that makes even more sense than the current, physical explanation for reality, and let us see how shifting our overall perspective of the Universe can deeply change the way we see ourselves.

Douglas Adams is a fabulous English writer who in 1978 brought us the book "Hitchhiker's Guide to the Galaxy." This wonderful science fiction parody is filled with truths and jokes alike, "Space, is big. Really big. You just won't believe how vastly, hugely, mindbogglingly big it is. I mean, you may think it's a long way down the road to the chemist's, but that's just peanuts to space." We laugh, but the fact is that anytime you stare up into the night sky, most every star and planet you see is in our neighborhood. The majority of the really faint ones are still in our own local galaxy, the Milky Way. That means that nearly everything we can see in the "vastness of space" with our naked eye is within ~30,000 light years. 30,000 light years just happens to be about the distance to the black hole at the center of the Milky Way. Our solar system sits out on one of the spiral arms of this amazing, spinning collection of 500 billion other stars.

If you live in a place far away from city lights as I do… and better, if you also have a pair of binoculars or a small telescope, you can see a faintly blurry "star" when you look just to the right of the Cassiopeia constellation. During late summer, she rises in a "W" shape in the Northern Hemisphere. What you are seeing is not a star, but in fact is another galaxy we call Andromeda. It's twice as big as our Milky Way and contains an estimated one trillion stars. It is the nearest large galaxy to us and it's about the only object you can see with your unaided eyes that's outside of our galaxy. This means that with the naked eye, we can just barely make out a something in space that is 2.5 million light years away. If you are fortunate to have a telescope, you'll be able to see that this tiny dot of Andromeda is actually just the brightest, center portion of an amazing spiral galaxy which appears six times larger than the full Moon but is too dim to see without magnification.

2.5 million light years away sounds really far away, but don't forget how we started off the chapter with that other galaxy 32 billion light years away. Trust me, in the not too distant future we will be finding galaxies that are twice that far away… think of the Saturn moon story.

Even with the vastness of space, scientists continue to calculate limits. They've tried to define the distance to the "edge" of the Universe, and they've even put a hard date on the "beginning" of the Universe. One thing that both science and mathematics abhor is the term "infinity." Truly, you will see them run for the cover of a mathematical constant in the attempt to avoid anything to do with the implications of infinity. The same goes for the term "energy" when you put matter in energetic terms. Everything in accepted science has to be finite, measurable, and tangible so that it concurs with the accepted knowledge-base and secures government grants for academics. Sad but true.

So lets toss those limits out. We really must check out the limitless horizon in a book titled, "The Qi Effect." Qi is life-force energy and by definition is without limits. If we are going to weave Qi into our cosmology story, we had better enter the realm of infinity.

According to Quantum Physicists, we are immersed in a quantum vibratory field effect. Quantum Physics holds that within that field of coherent energy, minute subatomic elements vibrate. In some theories, these subatomic elements are referred to as "Strings." The String Theory is a branch of Quantum Mechanics that attempts to explain the whole of our Universe up to a certain point, but it is basically a mathematics exercise and has pretty much been debunked. This includes all matter, dark matter, and waves. I agree with some of the discoveries emerging from these fields, but then again it's always been easy for me to accept that beyond all of the "strings" and "particles" lies a quantum flux of energetic vibrations and interference patterns. This is a tough one for physicists of any persuasion, and that's why these Quantum Physicists also find comfort in calling themselves Partical Physicists. It's fascinating how they just can't let go of "particles" or "strings" any more than a horder can get rid of their childhood collection of baseball cards or Barbie dolls.

I have no such attachments to physical or temporal domains, and so I am at ease with releasing the need for any tangible "thing" to stand in as "the fundamental" building block of the Universe. Practicing Qigong, Tai Chi, Yoga and Meditation makes it easy to accept intuitive insights into the fully energetic structure of the world around us at the deepest levels.

We've all seen those engaging animations that illustrate changes in visual scale. One that comes to mind pans across a single a strand of hair before suddenly zooming inside one of the hair cell's. Just as quickly, we increase magnification to see the protein molecule that makes up the cell. And then boom, the atoms that make up that protein molecule take center stage. Once we are inside the atom's electron cloud, we go on an incredibly long journey to get to the nucleus of the atom where we find dancing protons and neutrons. We continue increasing magnification until we see the the sub-atomic constituents of the sub-atomic particles known as quarks. The animation usually stop there because whew, that was amazing and exhausting to see just how complex a tiny strand of hair really is.

What happens if we magnify beyond the quarks? Will the conditioned scientific minds attempt to find yet an even tinier particle? At this point in time, science agrees that up quarks and down quarks make up protons and neutrons, and that the mass of every stable atomic nucleus is the most fundamental building block of matter. It is also agreed upon that quarks of any orientation or color cannot exist on their own, but can only be found when then come together in the form of protons and neutrons. At this level of granularity, I believe we've hit the edge of "particle" descriptions and really must come to accept that what we are really dealing with are energy fields. I'm doing my best to simplify the science here in order to paint a clear picture of how absurd it is not to accept our building blocks are in fact energy and not particles.

We just traveled to two limits that modern science has defined: the farthest reach of the Universe and the smallest resolution of the Universe. When there are spacial limits there must also be temporal limits, for this is the very definition of space and time.

Suppose for a moment the meaning of "infinity." What if truly infinite energetic vectors are the fundamental nature of our reality, both from the very large to the very small?

If we can operate from this "out of the space/time box" perspective, we can easily have a Universe that is "infinitely" old. All that really means is that the Universe has always existed and does so beyond the constraints of linear time. We can just as easily have a Universe that is "infinitely" large, extending in every direction infinitely. This idea naturally brings snickers from the scientific establishment as they quickly toss us calculations and theoretical models. Notice that they are "theoretical" models. Theoretical models can't prove a thing, they can only agree with other theories. If you do your research, you'll find that not all scientists agree with each other. So let's continue onward with our own "theory."

In a Universe that is allowed to express her infinite nature, there are no constraints on any "steady state" balance of matter and energy. In a truly infinite Universe, you have a lot more room (physicist call it "degrees of freedom") to explain what is currently unexplainable. There are actually many theories attempting to explain the "origin" of the Universe, the best contender being the Cyclical Universe Theory. The Cyclical Universe Theory is a bit of a hybrid Big Bang Theory that allows for many other smaller "bangs" to have occurred over much longer timespans. This theory emerged in 2002 out of Princeton University, and is notable because it explains many things that the current Big Bang theory cannot by introducing the existence of a 'parallel Universe.' Parallel to the Universe we live full of visible matter is another Universe filled with the life-force energy that is required to sustain ours.

This idea of parallel universes, one with matter and one with life-force energy, can be seen as another valid perspective one can take on viewing the "origin" story of our Universe. Mainstream science clings to a material perspective, evaluating time and space as finite and searching high and low for particulars to act as proof. Watching mainstream scientists repeatedly attempt to make sense out of only the things they have been conditioned to perceive is actually a bit sad. It's like a child crying in a sandbox because they've lost their favorite toy. They can't see it, but the toy is lying there just outside of the sandbox. In an infinite universe there is massive room for solutions to exist far beyond what anyone presently perceives, and as such, there may be simple ways to easily account for any calculations current science feels are out of balance with their perception. The whole concept of "balance" presupposes "finite space." To even begin to determine whether something is balanced or not, one must be able to see and measure all the parts and pieces in question. We think we can see the whole picture of the universe, when in fact we are really trapped inside of our five-senses' limited perception of the universe being finite. This is not much different than the exasperated child unable to perceive the limitless horizon of toys existing on both sides of the sandbox. We each have the choice to move beyond our concept of the finite and into the infinite. In the next chapter we'll discuss closed "containers" and open "conduits" in order to apply these concepts of the universe within our personal universe of body and mind.

The dimension of time works the same way. When we shift into perceiving the nature of our Universe as infinite, we no longer need to look to time to determine the "creation point" as we have done with the Big Bang. It is embedded within our ancient belief structure that just as each of us is born, everything including the Universe must also have an origin story. Emerging and groundbreaking research like the Doppler red-shift and "proof" of background noise in the Universe is conveniently mapped onto preconceived notions and are made to fit until at some point, it finally doesn't. This is important to the average person like you and me because our world views actually define the world we view. I learned that at University in Philosophy 101. If you want to be free, you've got to get out of your cage at every level. This is what the Qi Effect is all about. This

Universe has also always been here, experiencing star creation and black hole creation, star death and blackhole collapse. This is the fundamental nature of our Universe because it is the fundamental nature of this specific dimension. This particular reality is in constant chaotic flux, and that chaos drives creation at every level. It always has and always will.

Dimensions are not just a concept taken from science fiction, but they are a very basic part of quantum physics. In physics, the term "dimension" is used interchangeably with the term "degree of freedom." Some physicists conjecture that there are 11 distinct dimensions, though some String Theorists allow for 12 dimensions. I know this starts sounding a bit like science fiction, but this is indeed existing science and the mathematics required to justify it. The big question always is whether these "other dimensions" are observable. The subatomic elements, up-quarks, down-quarks, colors, etc., that make up our atoms appear to naturally move between dimensions. Apparently, it sounds more scientific when you say a subatomic element "expressed a new degree of freedom" than if you said that same subatomic element "moved into another dimension." The fact is, the two phrases mean the same thing and neither would give your Grandmother the warm fuzzies to hear that bits and pieces of her kitchen are in a constant state of interdimensional, energetic flux… The fact is that they are, but thankfully it is happening at such minute levels that Grandma can keep cooking dinner and her utensils don't disappear randomly…

To quote from An Introduction to Qigong Health Care: "There are many new fields of research including Systems Biology, Electrophysiology and Magnetogenetics that are starting to apply physics to biochemistry by defining the relationship between energy and physiology. Energy is being characterized as a flow of information. For example, researchers in the field of biofield physiology explore the information flow resulting from electromagnetic fields that living systems generate to regulate biological function and homeostasis. Other researchers are exploring the interconnections and exchanges between energy and information in the brain using cognitive and thermodynamic modeling." As Einstein described in his famous E=mc2 equation, there is a "relative relationship" between energy and mass, and the more we embrace this, the more we will begin to understand the QI Effect.

The concept of various dimensions are part of complex mathematical calculations that attempt to describe some of the amazing curiosities that occur during quantum-level events. Quantum-level events theoretically happen inside of stars and also at the edges of our Earth's atmosphere with the exposure of cosmic rays. The latest findings, of 2021 at the time of this writing come from the Event Horizon Telescope (EHT). The EHT is actually a consortium of the largest and best telescopes located around the Earth that all work together to act as a single enormous telescope looking at a combination of light, radio frequencies, x-rays, and infrared bandwidths. Combining these various frequencies into composite images allows us to get our first glimpses of a Black Hole. The most recent images are of a supermassive Black Hole which exists at the center of the nearby radio galaxy, Centaurus A. This Black Hole has a mass that is 55 million times that of our Sun and emits a jet of subatomic particles literally thousands of light years out from its Event Horizon. An Event Horizon is the "edge of no return" around a Black Hole where all matter, even light, is captured by the massive gravity that actually bends space and time. Over 100 years ago, Einstein correctly predicted in his General Relativity Theory that this warping of space/time was the very fabric of our reality. The international EHT team with their images of Centaurus A provide visual proof that subatomic particles "appear from some unexplainable source" and are sent far out into the Universe nearly at the speed of light on jets that defy current understanding. These new images have allowed us to finally see the "shadow" of an Event Horizon for the first time. We are beginning to realize how Black Holes play an alchemical role by constantly infusing the Universe with subatomic resources, the very building blocks of matter itself. As a result, Black Holes are constantly affecting and changing the nature of our dimension.

Back on Earth, inside particle accelerators like the one at CERN in Switzerland, physicists observe quantum effects that also defy our current understanding. Smash one atom against another at nearly the speed of light and amazing things take place. One curiosity is that new forms of the smashed atoms, radical waveform versions of unstable matter, are created and disappear. Although their existence lasts only for a tiny fraction of a second, their presence defies what we know about the world around us. Some subatomic particles seem to disappear while others seem to appear. This is where the mathematical necessity for multiple dimensions arises. When atoms are smashed, some subatomic particles go into another dimension. And where did the newly-appearing subatomic particles come from? Yes, they too came from another dimension. There is no other way to mathematically describe what is occurring other than to rely on the concept of "degree of freedom." In the quantum realm, many of these degree of freedom options entail "elements" simultaneously existing in not only another dimension, but everywhere at once. This is described in Schrödinger's Equation, which proves mathematically that on the quantum level of reality, there is a probability that matter can appear in multiple places at once. It is only in the presence of an observer that matter appears to be fixed to one location. Don't worry, Schrödinger neatly explains this wave function effect and thanks to probability factors, your next cup of tea will most likely not disappear in a puff of, well, improbability.

This stuff isn't made up, and it isn't written by Gene Roddenberry of Star Trek fame or George Lucas of Star Wars fame, though I have personally talked with both of them at length. This concept of multiple dimensions is in fact accepted by the most conservative and renowned physicists in the world. Dimensions other than the one we are currently experiencing is the only explanation for where these subatomic particles "disappear" to and emerge from whether this happens in particle accelerator experiments or in outer space.

Probably the most curious observation that fails to make sense to physicists who enjoy a neat and orderly materialistic view of the world is what is known as the "double slit" experiment. This is a process where either light, electrons, atoms, or even molecules are projected towards a metal plate that has two parallel slits cut into it. If everything was purely "matter," then everything projected would go through either one slit or the other. It's simple, one "thing" travels on one path. What is perplexing about this experiment, an experiment replicated and refined for over 200 years, is that the "matter" appears to pass through BOTH slits at the same time. This is shown through an "interference pattern" visible behind the metal plate. This phenomenon can be explained in two ways. Either matter can appear in two places at the same time, or things are not particles at all and are in fact energy waves. Thus, we have what is to this day known as the "wave-particle duality."

On a macro-scale, the most current observations of the Hubble Space Telescope clearly show high-resolution images of what Einstein's General Theory of Relativity describe as "gravitational lensing." These images show light from galaxies billions of light years away being warped by the massive gravitational fields that exist around giant galaxies and Black Holes. What is amazing is that this is not just an optical effect like you would see through a wavy piece of glass. Space/time itself is being stretched and warped by gravity. This means that in many locations throughout our Universe, what we consider "normal and consistent" reality is very far from normal and consistent. Our idea of a fixed dimension is put into question by the most intelligent minds in science.

The scientific community has an ultimate need for alternative dimensions because they satisfy the complex mathematical calculations and account for the "everything else" that occurs in these types of high-speed, particle collision experiments. Alternative dimensions also explain pretty much everything in the farthest reaches of space.

So why is the scientifically proven existence of alternative dimensions relevant in a book on Qi?

Well, the most important reason is that Qi actually doesn't reside in this dimension. This life-force, life-sustaining energetic component plays a vital role in our world and yet it doesn't exist in the same dimension that your body does. It doesn't reside in this observable physical world at all, which is why Qi has never been seen or measured, and why we only recognize its effect. The field of quantum physics and the emerging field of Quantum Biology, which I will get into later on in this book, have helped bridge the ideas of the ancients by scientifically confirming that Qi exists even if it doesn't reside in our dimension. Thousands of years ago, medicine and the healing arts belonged to the domain of mystics and spiritual elders. They saw the body along with the entire material world through an energetic perspective where everything is interwoven and interrelated. They understood the massive influence an observer has on illness, and they recognized and used the power of sound, including chants, music, mantras, incantations, etc., to facilitate healing. What they knew intuitively is exactly what quantum physics and quantum biology principles are proving to be true. Qi absolutely influences our dimension and everything in it in ways that ancient healers and mystics knew by living with one foot in the material world and the other in the world of energy.

Imagine "empty" space... that vast and amazing expanse of darkness that goes on for tens of trillions of miles in light years between stars and planets. We use "empty" with quotes because we know now that space is anything but empty. Not only is there a quantum vibratory field and universal "background noise" present everywhere in "empty" space, but there is also what science is calling "dark matter" and "dark energy." I won't go to deep into astrophysics, but I will say that mainstream science is absolutely clear that not a single cubic centimeter of space anywhere in the Universe is empty. It was Einstein who is attributed to saying that any cubic centimeter, about the size of a pea, holds the potential energy to power a whole city. Nobel Laureate Michael Faraday originated the theory that all of reality is made up of "lines of force." His theory predicts that electricity, light, and gravity are all related energetics. One hundred years later, Einstein wrote the equation that linked energy with mass, showing they are interchangeable and in a dynamic relationship. Not long after Einstein, the age of atomic energy began putting his theories into action. Soon after, Nicolai Tesla and Galileo Ferrara applied similar concepts by creating power generators that we currently use today to power our standard alternating current (AC) electrical system.

We have vast regions of the Universe appearing as empty space where suddenly "nothing" become something. Einstein famously showed us how matter could not be created or destroyed. He also proved that energy and matter were interchangeable. The great darkness of outer space is infused with massive amounts of energy in which the elegant transition of energy into matter is taking place. Energy transforms into matter to various extents everywhere, all of the time. It is only because of our limited senses and technology that we think this exchange is restricted to molecular clouds and nebulae.

Science agrees that hydrogen is the most abundant "matter" in the Universe. Hydrogen means "the smallest stable atom possible." And that's what it is: one electron, one proton, and one neutron. You can't be smaller than that and still be an atom because atoms require all three aforementioned subatomic particles. So it makes sense that hydrogen would be the most abundant component in the Universe since it's the most simple. Because of its ultimate simplicity, Hydrogen is the first "matter" to emerge from the incredible transformation of energy into matter.

This is what this dimension of our Universe does: it transforms energy into matter. All of the fabulous hydrogen-filled nebulae and molecular clouds strewn across the Universe are evidence of this and are typically the places where stars are born. Stars too are composed mainly of Hydrogen.

If everything, including the stars, are made up of Hydrogen, the logical next step is to inquire into where all of this Hydrogen is coming from. Hydrogen transitions slowly from tiny subatomic particles (electrons, up-quarks, and down-quarks) that dance into this physical dimension through the transformative flow of energy into matter. The reason mainstream science claims Hydrogen to be the first and smallest component of the Universe to exist is simply because it is the first and smallest thing that we can "see." Just because our limited senses and technology cannot look out into space and "see" subatomic particles does not mean they are not there.

Science hasn't yet grasped that in our incredibly life-force charged Universe, the transition from the chaotic, quantum field of energy morphing into subatomic elements is happening all the time. Energy, expressed as electro-magnetic fields in our dimension, "congeals" with elegantly intelligent coherence into subatomic elements throughout the Universe. This is what energy in this dimension appears to naturally do. Energy changes states and frequencies until various coherent vibrations, known as interference patterns, align. When this occurs, a "subatomic particle" that corresponds to that coherent vibration comes into existence. It's not that it is created, it simply is a change in state, no different on some level than the way gas turns into water and water turns into ice. In the same way, for energy/matter transformation, energy moves from the quantum field flux vibration to become what we call quarks. The quarks then gain coherence and congeal into protons, neutrons, electrons, electron neutrinos, and others curious subatomic members that are simply distinguished based on charge, frequency, and density. The dance known as "strong forces," is similar to gravity but actually much stronger. During "strong forces," the three largest and most stable subatomic elements (protons, neutrons, and electrons) find their next most basic, stable, and highest probable combination: the simplest atomic matrix we call Hydrogen.

It may also be interesting to note the the most abundant molecule in our body is water. We all can say we "know" that water makes up 70% of our body… but in fact 95% of the molecules in our body are water molecules. Water is denoted as H_2O because it is made up on Hydrogen and Oxygen, actually twice as many Hydrogen atoms as Oxygen atoms. If Hydrogen is truly the bridge between energy and matter, rest assured that your body is living proof of an energy matrix expressing the Qi Effect.

This transition from energy-to-matter is taking place all the time and has gone on since infinity. It is key to how our bodies, grow, heal, and rejuvenate. It is fundamental to how stars and matter itself come into being. We don't need a Big Bang to explain how the Universe that we see all around us came into being. Explanations of origin theories have simply been a ploy to keep us trapped into a self-limiting, materialistic view of our world.

The ancient Chinese Taoists didn't have a Big Bang per se, although they did embrace the idea that at one time there was only the Wuji, or the void. This is what modern science would say existed before the Bang itself. Out from the Wuji emerged the undifferentiated "One" called Yuan Qi. To me, this "One" points to the quantum field itself. The Taoists continue that from the One came the Two (huang ji): Yin and Yang. Yin and Yang are the observable complimentary energies that seem to be everywhere in our dimension, such as positive and negative forces. This parallels the first subatomic elements emerging into this dimension with negatively charged electrons and positively charged protons. Note that the up quarks and down quarks are yet just another reflection of the ubiquitous, complementary nature of Yin and Yang.

The Taoist view continues, noting that from the Two came the Three. Different Taoists interpret this in different ways. Within every atom, aside from positively and negatively charged particles, there is a neutron with a neutral charge. The Three can refer to the interrelationship that occurs when subatomic particles first unite to create atoms. The first and most simple expression of this, as previously discussed, is the atom we call Hydrogen. Ancient Chinese Taoists refer to Yuan Qi, or the "primordial life-force" as what emerges from the Wuji emptiness to start the creation process. It is believed that this Yuan Qi is the "neutral" energetic joining "negative" Yin and "positive" Yang to form the Three at this stage of the creation process.

Next, the Taoist cosmology observes as the Three transforms into the Five. There was no need for the Four as this was more about essence unfolding than a math logic exercise. The Five are the five basic elements (wu xing) of the physical world. To the Taoist, these elements are Wood, Fire, Earth, Metal and Water. Again, these are symbolic metaphors that serve well as a language to explain many things. For our Qi Effect perspective on cosmology, we can look at the Five as those five basic Taoist elements and then relate them to all the elements that are formed inside every star.

Finally, the Five gives way to the Ten Thousand, as Lao Tzu laid out in Taoism's core text, the "Tao de Ching". This naturally refers to everything in the material world. All of the elements that emerge from within the stars come together in the incredible ways they do to form everything we see around us from the planets to our bodies.

I don't believe that the ancient Taoists were suggesting the above process happened in a single moment of creation, but in fact, in their genius, they were describing what takes place constantly in the creation of matter through the transition of energy-to-matter. They precisely intuited what takes place both in the far reaches of outer space and inside every atom of your body.

It appears that the "origin of everything" laid out above corroborates with not only the structure of quantum physics, but also the amazing intuition the Taoists expressed in the language of Qi over 2,500 years ago. You may ask whether this quantum background energy in our universe is the same as Qi? Good question.

In my perspective, the answer is No.

Well then, why did I take you down this long path only to negate Qi? Isn't this book was supposed to be about Qi?

We actually didn't negate Qi at all. We just haven't explored the process that quantum background energy undergos in order to transition into the subatomic particles we call quarks and electrons. We haven't yet understood where the energy comes from that allows this incredible transformation to occur.

It's all thanks to Qi.

No one can prove if I am right or wrong because there is actually no solid proof for any of the current widely accepted theories. If you stay connected to your intuition as you follow the logic I am about to lay before you, you may realize that the concept of the Qi Effect makes a lot of sense. It can shift many things you've been wondering about: the power of intention, spontaneous healing, and even how life is created and sustained.

Inside the quantum physicists' subatomic accelerator laboratories, subatomic particles appear and disappear, seemingly moving in and out of dimensions. What is happening inside of these highly controlled experiments is exactly what is happening all of the time throughout the entire Universe. My sense is that it's not just happening in massive nebulae where hydrogen gas clouds many light-years wide are forming stars. It's happening in every atom, in every molecule, in every cell of your body.

The transformation of energy into matter is taking place all around us all of the time. If this is true, then the reciprocal must be happening as well: matter is continually being transformed into energy. This process of transformation only makes sense as a cycle going in both directions, otherwise the homestasis and stability we experience in this Universe would not be able to be sustained. The energy-to-matter transition process is what creates subatomic particles that enter our dimension (infinitesimally small, Planck-sized waveforms that merge with our atoms). The matter-to-energy process accounts for subatomic particles "leaving" this dimension, as is curiously demonstrated in the quantum physicists' subatomic accelerator laboratories. These are subtle energy fluxes that happen so harmoniously and naturally inside every atom that for the most part we don't even notice it in everyday life. But without it, life and the very structure of reality would most likely not exist. We will come to eventually discover that this process is what sustains atoms as the dynamic and vital energetic structures they are. It is also part of what keeps our bodies animated and alive. Just because science hasn't yet measured this does not mean that it's not true.

The big question remains: what initiates and sustains this interdimensional transfer of subatomic, energetic waveforms? The answer is simply Qi.

Qi is the life-force energy that the ancient Taoists intuited. They, like the ancients of many cultures, "knew" there was a force of some kind sustaining life. Albeit elusive, it seemed possible to cultivate through various practices. It appears to occur abundantly and naturally when we are young, and sometimes it expresses itself spontaneously. People have always said it's all around us even though we can't see it or measure it. We can feel it, though. This is a very wonderful, romantic and poetic point of view that makes Qi out to be very mystical indeed. Acupuncturists and energy healers actually believe that they can "move" Qi, especially if it is blocked or stagnant. Others believe that they can send you their Qi. I will address these most curious ideas in another chapter. For now, I will say that from my perspective Qi is not in our dimension whatsoever, while its influence is absolutely all around us. Currently, there is no biochemical theory or observation that can explain what sustains life. Science can describe all of the complex processes down to mitosis, mitochondria, and the ATP Cycle, but they can't explain what kicks off the process and what sustains it. The life-force energy behind all we see remains elusive.

Precisely how subatomic waveforms, or particles, move in and out of our dimension is the key to understanding Qi's role in "matter." What happens to "matter" in the process of coming in and out of existence in our dimension? The most fundamental explanations in quantum physics account for this in Schrödinger's Equation, Hilbert Space, quantum entanglement, and quantum tunneling. We will discuss each of these further in the next chapter.

Qi plays a powerfully energetic role by catalyzing subatomic waveforms and providing them with what is required to "jump dimensions." Einstein's core work with E=mc2 explores the dynamic relationship between energy and matter. Woven together with quantum principles, it shows how Qi fits into our reality. Subatomic waveforms, such as electrons and quarks, are actually energetic quantum of vibratory fields. They can change their pattern and field effect in such a way as to slip from a known locations in this dimension into another. Many times they appear in multiple locations at once. More importantly, they tunnel into another "degree of freedom." This "degree of freedom" is the dimension where Qi resides.

Many great minds have contributed to the support of this concept. During dawn of Quantum physics, in the early 1900's, the German mathematician David Hilbert developed an array of conceptual maps for mathematically projecting 3-dimensional space into essentially infinitely-dimensional space. This is the only way to help understand and explain what is being observed in the minute quantum realm of reality and in this sense "dimension" is more about energetic information that physical, Euclidean 3D space. These theoretical models demonstrate how subatomic waveforms can assume infinite-dimensional spaces, and have been corroborated by research conducted decades later in the aforementioned atom smashers. High-speed particle accelerators show us that bits and parts of atoms really do appear and disappear, defying logic and classical physics. Each passing year in science brings more questions than answers, yet what we keep discovering is that our world is much more amazing than we ever expected.

Our timeless and infinite Universe has been dancing into this dimension we call home forever. We perceive The Universe through our five senses in its material form as the world we live in. What we aren't aware of is that the Universe is undergoing many transformational stages in the quantum field and is constantly being energized by Qi. We will refer to this as the Qi Field. The Qi Field provides the necessary energy to bring The Universe into being through quantum tunneling subatomic waveforms. These subatomic waveforms naturally form into their first coherent atomic relationship, Hydrogen. Eventually enough Hydrogen pulls together by successively increasing gravitational attraction over hundreds of thousands of years, and a young star is born. Yes, that's how all stars are formed. All 500 billion stars in our Milky Way, including our Sun, all of the one trillion stars in Andromeda, and every one of the infinite of galaxies dancing throughout our Universe.

Eventually every star, like every living being, reaches the end of its life cycle. This can be anywhere from a few million years to many billions of years. The oldest star we are currently aware of is around 14 billion years old which is older than the Universe itself, which is supposed to be about 13.8 billion years old. This is just more proof that the Big Bang and the "creation" of the Universe doesn't really make sense.

Let us take a closer look at one of these elder stars. A star getting on it ints year, like our Sun, will reach the end part of it's life being primarily made up of hydrogen, the simplest known atomic manifestation to emerge from the energetic quantum field. What makes a star shine is the Hydrogen burning as fuel in the fusion reaction that takes place inside of every star. Over time, the star begins to contain Helium. Helium is the second smallest physical manifestation to emerge from the energetic quantum field. Can you see the pattern? Stars are the visible transformation of energy into matter. Of course we won't witness rocking chairs or cell phones popping out of the quantum field because the transformation occurs in gradual stages as the dial slowly turns from "energy" towards "matter." Doesn't this make sense? Matter is made up of atoms and atoms are all neatly arranged in the Table of Elements based on their mass, structural complexity, and essentially, their vibratory frequency. This Table always made me think of musical notation as each atom had its own harmonic tone and when these various elements are combined, it is a bit like a symphony were the whole is greater than the sum of its parts. Elements created within a star become denser and more complex as that star begins to die and collapse and it plays out its final cosmic symphony.

In that elder star that is entering its final stage of life, Hydrogen has burned up and its supply has run out. Massive heat and gravitational collapse begins as the transformation from subatomic particles into Hydrogen intensifies into Helium. Helium follows suit and both elements create core rings inside the star, similar to the layers of an onion. The massive heat and gravitational conditions inside a collapsing, exploding star gives rise through atomic fusion reactions to creating increasingly larger, denser, and more complex atoms. Typically, when the heavy Iron atom is created, the end of that star is at hand and with it arrives the creation of the myriad elements that make up our material world. The Earth, planets, moons, asteroids, and comets all come into being in this dimension through the aggregation of those star-created elements. It's actually quite amazing that it takes a dying star to spawn the physical world as we know it. Every single atom inside of our bodies originated inside of these stars that gave its life for us a very long, long time ago.

"Mother Nature" is thus not separate from "Humankind." That can be tough to accept, as we have been conditioned to see the two as separate and typically at odds with each other. Interchangeable, one is blamed for negatively affecting the other. At the same time, we talk about humans living in harmony with nature. The fact is that we all come from the same atoms. The energetic source is the same for the rocks and plants as the human body. We all are affected by the Sun and Moon, whether it's the way sunlight helps our bodies generate Vitamin D or the way the lunar gravity affects the ocean tide or a woman's monthly cycle. As long as we focus on the "difference" between nature and humans we will obscure our potential for seeing the "singularity." When we do accept the wider lens of "singularity," our world will exist in much sweeter harmony. No, it will not be perfect, for that's not the within the design-plan of this 3D experience it seems. Life can, however, be a much different and more harmonious experience for both Mother Earth and Humans. It all depends on energy and how we perceive it. The only place to begin is within our own bodies, our own minds, our emotions, our lifestyle, our community...

The goddess-worshipping, mystery school of Ancient Greece was based in Metaponto, now Southern Italy, and is where my paternal family-line originated. I've been there many times and have loads of beautiful family there. Many of them live in houses that have been in our family for literally hundreds of years. The most famous "priest" of this school is actually someone who I will gladly bet you studied in school: The amazing Greek, Pythagoras. In Italian we call him by the Romanized name "Pitagora," but it's the same person. Most likely in the eighth grade, we are taught that Pythagoras was a great mathematician who figured out how to calculate the unknown side of a right triangle, giving us what we call The Pythagorean Theorem. Architects love this equation because it makes it easy to problem-solve the layout of a floorpan. The fact is, math was probably the least of the many worthwhile artifacts old Pythagoras left us. As the head of a Goddess cult, he was the spiritual leader for many, many people. He was an astrologer, astronomer, healer, teacher, sacred-space developer, musician, and more. For a person like him, Mathematics was part and parcel of his vast understanding and served mainly to weave sacred geometry into every aspect of life. What I love most about him was his school motto, "We are the children of the stars."

How could he state this so clearly 2,600 years ago when we are only now understanding the astronomical origins of matter?

For the people who lived in the era of Pythagoras, before the Intellectual Mind was given such ability to shut down our Intuitive Mind, they trusted the wisdom that was within them. They understood the role of the unseen energies around them as a critical part of both themselves and the physical world they interacted with each day. The word "atom" was already a part of Greek vocabulary even though they had no electron microscopes. The word "pneuma" was also in their vocabulary to describe the life-force energy that infuses all things. The mystical philosophers of those days, much like their Taoist contemporaries in China, understood that the physical world we experience emerged from the ethers, fed by a life-giving energy that sustains this physical world. Of course in their view of the world, this life-force sustaining energy was attributed to various gods and the realms that they were responsible for. This way of thinking had been passed down for thousands of years before them, originating in the pre-Babylonian cultures of Sumer, Akkadia, and before in the Fertile Crescent of Mesopotamia. With the discoveries of places like Gobekli Tempe near the Turkey/Syria border, we now know that there were thriving cultures even thousands of years before that. Carbon-dated to 9,000 B.C.E., which is over 11,000 years ago, this massive and advanced temple complex predates the oldest writing in cuneiform by 5,000 years. What did those peoples know that has since been lost? What we can be quite certain of, based on core samples taken recently in Arctic glaciers, is that there was in fact a great flood that most likely occurred around 11,600 years ago. With it, a great many knowledges of the Universe were lost.

The knowledge that has been lost on a literal and material level is still innately within us in a deep and intuitive place. We all get glimpses from time to time that the world around us is not what it appears to be, yet we have been deeply conditioned to believe that what we see is all there is. It makes a good work force when people keep their nose to the grindstone, consumed with thoughts of survival. We have been trained to survive and not necessarily to "thrive." We have been convinced that "thriving" means upgrading to a bigger car or a fancier television by having more money. The meaning of "thrive" has been continually reshaped as our cultural belief systems steadily shift away from spiritual and energetic truth. We have been conditioned to embrace order and rules, and to see chaos negatively and as "disorder."

Imagine a time when chaos was seen as the creative force of the Universe. Imagine Chaos as a very good and positive friend only when you knew how to make peace and recognize her as a fundamental driver of the Universe. The ancient mystics knew Chaos as a powerful force and used her to great advantage. They knew that Chaos was the one who called "matter" out from the Great Void and into this physical dimension. The transformational role of Chaos mirrors the way that subatomic components attract and combine to form Hydrogen as well as how Hydrogen atoms cluster together to form stars. This alchemy is taking place everywhere around us, and the ancient Taoists knew this well on an intuitive and poetic level.

To truly understand the ancient Chinese Taoist mind and worldview on Qi, we need to go deep into the essence of how they saw and embraced chaos in their cosmology and in their alchemical approach to philosophy and healthcare.

One of the most mystical words and concepts emerging from ancient China, besides "Wuji", is "Hùndùn". Wuji represents the energetic "space" of our Infinite Universe, and literally translates to the "edge or limit of non-beingness." This is a fabulous, complex, and ancient concept that I will address at another time. Hundun, as a mystical complement to Wuji, is more of a dynamic process or quality that could be translated as "chaos." It is written 混沌. Understanding the essence of Hundun is not only fundamental to grasping the core concept of Qigong, but dramatically shifts the way we look at the world around us as well as how we perceive healing our body, mind, and spirit. Everything, from cutting-edge research in Quantum Mechanics to Epigenetics, makes references that can be traced back to the ancient concept of Hundun in one way or another. To understand the way that Hundun is woven into the very fabric of life will ask you to bring yourself into deep sensitivity with your personal development, the evolution of mankind, and the Universe itself.

"Hùn" traditionally translates as "chaos, muddled, or confused," carrying a relatively negative connotation. Over the centuries, Chinese classical texts have used Hundun with a variety of subtle yet distinct shades of meaning. In the classic Taoist classic "Zhuangzi," Hùn is written using a modified Chinese character ⼚ to signify "abundantly flowing; turbid water; torrent; mix up," and imbues it with an intention much more in line with Taoist philosophy. The character ⼚ also suggests the "sound of running water; confused." The expression "something confused and yet complete" (hun cheng) is found in the Dao de Jing 25 (Tao te Ching). Hun Cheng references the dynamic state that existed prior to the formation of the physical Universe. This pre-universe Universe contained a lifeforce of creation and an energetic intelligence where nothing was yet perceptible. This idea of an Infinite Consciousness was linked to the idea of a Universal Qi Field and wasn't simply the state "prior" to the physical world, but was in fact a fundamental dynamic of life that is ubiquitously present even in this very moment.

The ancient Taoists embraced the time "before" the physical Universe, the great infinite-potential state of Wuji from which all matter emerged. This "creation story" is accepted in Chinese culture and can provide insight into their cultural attitudes and norms. To the modern Chinese mind, it is a fundamental given that life will be chaotic and turbulent when control and order are not substantially imposed. This attitude stems from ancient Confucian attitudes, which were at odds with the Taoists of their time, and succeeded in creating a massive set of rules and edicts that influence Chinese thinking and culture to this day.

Hundun is written with the semantic "water radical" 水 or 氵 plus the phonetic "Kūn" 昆 and "Tún" 屯. Hundun as "primordial chaos" is a cognate of and etymologically related to "Huntun" 餛飩, ⼚ ⼚ "wonton; dumpling soup" written with the "eat" radical 食. The word we know in English as "Wonton" is borrowed from the Cantonese pronunciation "Wantan" and relates hundun and wonton, and refers to the "undifferentiated soup of primordial chaos." When energy begins to differentiate, dumpling-like blobs of matter coalesce out of the chaos. Note how similar this is to hydrogen being created out of the "emptiness" of space...

The English word chaos is associated with the translation of Hundun in a clearer way when you look at the classical sense of "Khaos" used in ancient Greek mythology, "gaping void; formless primordial space preceding creation of the Universe." The Greeks planted the seeds of Western philosophy from this perspective of the Universe. In modern times we associate "disorder and confusion" with chaos when actually this was not at all what the Ancient Greek or Chinese wisdom held to be true. Chaos did not hold a negative connotation, but in fact was a very positive, empowered concept. Chaos was understood to be a latent energy of creation with infinite potential, permeating everything including every atom in our bodies.

In all of the Confucian texts, the powerful and esoteric word Hundun was only used three times! The concept of an empowering Chaos was completely counter to the massively rule-based, controlling principles of Confucianism that claimed a rigid idea of"civilization." For the Confucians, there was no room for "infinite potential;" the only way to control people and society was by the way of a well-defined social and political structure defined by laws and norms.

Around 500 BCE, the Taoists were diametrically opposed to the Confucians. There is a story about the Confucian disciple Zigong being dumbfounded after meeting a Daoist Sage. When he reported back to Confucius, Confucius denigrated the Taoist by saying, "Hundun shi zhi shu." In English this translates to, "Those miserable arts of Mr. Chaos [Mr. Hundun]. Mr. Chaos is one of those bogus practitioners of the arts. He knows the first thing but doesn't understand the second. He looks after what is on the inside but doesn't look after what is on the outside." You can imagine how a rigid and intellectual Confucian concerned with outer appearances would be so utterly confused by the Taoist, Qigong-practicing Mr. Chaos.

The ancient Taoists embraced Hundun deeply because it explains how each of us who practice "the arts" like Qigong, Yoga, or Tai Chi are able to understand our true essence and access the healing and rejuvenating life-force of Qi. It seems that through accepting chaos in our lives, whether it appears as illness or conflict, our practice teaches us to flow with it, to learn from it, and to stay open to healing and transformation through it. In ancient times, these arts were called by names such as Shu Lian and Dao Yin. There are many, many other names for practices that were more shamanic in nature and focused on spiritual cultivation. They all sprouted from this core concept of dancing harmoniously through the Hundun and activating Qi in the proces.

Unlike the Confucian texts, Hundun commonly occurs in the classics of philosophical Taoism. The "Tao Te Ching" (Dao De Jing) does not mention Hundun directly but uses Hùn graphic variants. One section (49, tr. Mair 1990:17) uses hun ("bemuddle"): "The Sage is self-effacing in his dealings with all under heaven, and bemuddles his mind for the sake of all under heaven." Three others (14, 15, 25, tr. Mair 1990:74, 76, 90) use hun "bound together," "muddled," and "featureless" as follows:

"These three cannot be fully fathomed, Therefore, They are bound together to make unity."

"Plain, as an unhewn log, muddled, as turbid waters, expansive, as a broad valley."

"There was something featureless yet complete, born before Heaven and Earth."

Notice how in this case, "bemuddle" is used positively, referring to letting go of intellectual rigidity and the preconceived belief systems that have "programmed" us to lose sight of our innate, intuitive, Heart-mind wisdom.

Chuang Zi was a later contemporary of Lao Tzu and a renowned Taoist wizard with a clever wit. The aforementioned book "Chuangzi" (3rd-2nd centuries BCE) is attributed to him, containing a famous parable involving one Emperor Hundun, Emperor Shu 儵 (literally the name of a type of fish suggesting an 'abrupt; quick' attitude), and Emperor Hu 忽 (which translates to 'ignore; neglect; sudden'). Chuang Zi makes a joke comparing Emperor Hundun (the obvious Taoist) with two other Emperors caught up in common foibles of the intellectually-trapped, control-obsessed Confucian mind.

Two other Chuang Zi texts have a noteworthy use of hundun. One of them is an allegorical story about a man named Hong Meng 鴻蒙 "Silly Goose," who "was amusing himself by slapping his thighs and hopping around like a sparrow." The comparative religions scholar Norman Girardot interprets this action as "a type of shamanic dancing comparable with the Shanhaijing"(1983:110). Hong Meng poetically repeats the phrase "hunhun-dundun" to mean "dark and undifferentiated chaos" as he practices this Taoist "mind-nourishment" meditation technique. Here is another precursor of Qigong practice described to be quite "silly" to the uninitiated.

There were ancient Hundun-centered "Creation myths" in Chinese cosmology suggesting that life emerged from primordial chaos. This is so curiously in line with theories of modern Quantum Physics. There were also Shamanic Taoist chants and dances performed to evoke this primal state of mind. The word "Qigong" did not exist in ancient times, these practices were the precursors to what we now know as Qigong.

The world-system "hun tian" in ancient Chinese astronomy conceptualized the Universe as a round egg and the Earth as a yolk swimming within it. "Pangu" 盤古 is the mythological creator of the Universe who grew into a giant in order to separate Heaven and Earth. Heaven and earth as marital partners within the world-egg refers to the theme of Sky Father and Earth Mother goddess creating the Cosmic Egg... "Jie hun" is the Mandarin word for "marriage."

Hundun, used as a word to signify "primordial chaos," is key to "Neidan," Chinese internal alchemy. Wuji Hundun Qigong is a style of Qigong that I learned from Master Duan Zhi Liang, and has components of Neidan practice in its use of specific forms and movements to align our body and energy field (Wei Qi) with the essential "chaotic" nature of the Universe in order to overcome stagnation and activate vitality. It is through the embrace of Hundun that it is believed we can tap into and activate the original life-force Qi of creation for our health and rejuvenation. Thus, the primordial chaos of Hundun is the underlying, driving influence on Qi, and Qi is the life-force energetic behind all things dancing throughout the infinite, undifferentiated Wuji. To the ancient Taoists, Wuji might equate with the quantum background resonance throughout the whole of the Universe. The combination of Hundun within the Wuji, empowered by Qi, accounts for the creation of sub-atomic particles and atoms themselves, consciousness itself, and the animation of all living things.

The rebel philosopher Heraclitus of Ancient Greece famously said, "The only thing constant is change." What is more chaotic than constant change? Just as every atom is created from an accumulation of chaotic subatomic elements infused by Qi, each individual consciousness, whether human, animal, or plant, is pulled out from the infinite consciousness and infused by Qi. In its essence, consciousness is just another quantum field coherence emerging out of our Universe's wave function. As the ancients of many cultures sensed, virtually everything is conscious and animate to one degree or another. It might actually be the chaos in the quantum energy field that initiates and the triggers probability for consciousness to emerge.

Chaos Theory is actually a formal path of study in mathematics and is applied to fields including material physics, quantum physics, biology, meteorology, encryptology, robotics, DNA computing, social behavior, and economics. Eventually all fields will encompass some level of Chaos Theory to better understand the essence of that field and to help develop predictive models as that's what this path of calculation is really all about – predicting outcomes.

It is a time-honored dream to know what will happen in the future and what could be more desirous to calm our deepest survival fears than to know the outcome of current choices and conditions. This is the basis of Chaos Theory as it recognizes that most all situations carry some level of chaos, or unpredictability yet it poses that if you can fully understand current conditions and possible influences, you can deduce a high probability for the most likely outcome. Well, knowing that this type of predictive analytics is applied heavily in weather forecasting, we know that it's an imperfect science… go ask anyone who picked a beach day based on the weather reports only to have it rain on a supposed sunny day.

The fact is, Chaos Theory shows quite conclusively that even within the chaotic structure of any system (from weather to economics) there is a certain level of high probability outcomes that – with enough good data, including historic patterns – will get you close to knowing what may unfold.

Humans are curious creatures that so want to calm their fears and have some handle on the future. Whether it was the ancient Etruscans who had their wise ones who could read auguries in the livers of animals, or the famed Oracle of Delphi in Greece who would be consulted by great generals and kings, our desire to know the future by reading signs in the present is a basic survival drive. We all do it in one way or another and we all recognize the role of life's chaotic nature that reminds us how difficult it is to really know what will occur even in the near future.

Henri Poincaré, the French mathematician and physicist, was the first who really defined chaotic deterministic systems. His breakthrough calculations relating to chaotic probabilities of gravitational waves in 1905 influenced the great minds of the time including Einstein and Poincaré's concepts helped him lead to his own theory of relativity that came out soon thereafter. I guess you could have predicted that...

Heartbeat rhythms and eye movements of schizophrenic patients were later discovered to be chaotic movements and followed deterministic chaotic trajectories, which means that they were not just random. Complex adaptive, non-linear systems are really a fancy way of describing the human body. It is important to understand the difference between random and chaotic since chaos infers certain order and some guiding force at work.

This is the part I really like because it brings up two important thoughts... First, the work of Illya Prigogine who won the Nobel Prize for evolving systems. He proved at the point of perturbation (chaos) that they don't decay into some entropic mess, but rather, they move to a new, higher level of order. The second thought of course is the Qi Effect itself.

What is this driving force within chaos that evolves systems – like our body and the body politic – to higher levels of order? Could this be the activation of Qi lifeforce energy as described in the Qi Effect? How is it that there is a level of intelligence at work that defies logic and just when you think things will fall apart and get worse, they actually attain a new level order out of the apparent chaos. What's even better is that the Qi Effect reminds us – as does Quantum Physics – that you, the observer – has a massive influence over this outcome.

It is a futile attempt to predict very specific outcomes, and Chaos Theory also defines the impossibility of doing so the farther out in time you go. It's easy to relate this to meteorological weather forecasts or the prediction of stock prices on Wall Street. Nonetheless, spontaneous order emerges out of chaos and the theory claims that this is triggered by strange attractors, whatever they may be. Don't worry, even Einstein fretted over this one. Whether it is a crystalline structure growing in nature or evolving social system dynamics, something drives this order out of chaos besides force of biochemical reactions or individual intention. Could this be the role of Qi?

It was our favorite Taoist, Chuang Zi in the 4th Century BC who discussed that when systems or social orders were simply left alone, the energetic force of nature (the Tao) would always allow for spontaneous order. This is why so many of us who like holistic energy healing, small government, and Libertarianism deeply relate to Taoism. Conflicting differences and emergent behaviors amongst large groups of people actually lead to spontaneous dynamic order in Chaos Theory. This shows that fascist control and censorship is actually the wrong approach if you truly seek natural and harmonious order. This is precisely why Chuang Zi turned away from the central power-oriented Confucians at the time... Hmm... maybe some things really don't change after all...

Back in the late '70s when my first elder energy-healing teacher passed, I went on to study with one of his long-time students, Barbara Marx Hubbard. It was then that I was reintroduced to Hundun from a very Western perspective. I am most grateful to Barbara for taking me into her world and introducing me to her and her partner John Whiteside's inner circle of spiritual and political leaders. Amongst the luminaries with whom I shared meals and lengthy conversations, from Gene Roddenberry of Star Trek to the Karmapa Lama of Tibet, was that aforementioned Nobel Laureate named Ilya Prigogine. Ilya, a Russian-born Belgian, had recently won a Nobel Prize in Chemistry (1977). Prompted by my youthful curiosity, Ilya kindly explained what exactly he won his Nobel prize for. In the middle of telling me his story, he revealed that his prize winning discoveries about chlorine molecules were just a front. He and his team of graduate students had been mainly focused on spiritual matters. I was hooked. He leaned in and explained his basic theory that can be summed up as all biologically evolving systems have to reach a point of maximum perturbation before they attain their next higher level of order. Perturbation simply means chaos, hundun incarnate. He said that science had misconceived entropy, the process of decay, and that we actually are all constantly evolving to higher and higher levels of order. To fully appreciate Ilya's theory, we have to embrace the chaotic nature of the process, and essentially make peace with it.

If we are to embrace this process whose nature is essentially one of chaos, we may begin to wonder what, if anything, is behind the chaos. What sustains the Wuji quantum wave function, and for that matter, what empowers Qi itself?

I feel that these are personal questions, questions that each of us needs to reflect upon on a regular basis. They are like the unanswerable Zen Koans. We take them inside and simply allow them to sit in our Heart resonance, embraced by our Intuitive Mind. We don't seek a specific answer as we simply remain receptive to what we receive. This is the spiritual journey.

Typically, the practical level of the Mind reaches two conclusions:

1) It can all be explained scientifically, there is nothing behind life and creation that lies outside of quantification

2) A Creator of Infinite Consciousness permeates everything

How and what you choose is up to you; no one but you can tell you what is so. This is the beauty of our life journey. At the depth of our being we accept our sense of how life is created and sustained, and we dance in the miracle that unfolds around us. To be settled and at peace about our personal belief around the process of life itself allows us to honor the miraculous process of birth and accept the inevitable and equally miraculous process of death. If we look for it, we can find that it also gives us a particular grounding and understanding of all that occurs between, before, and after, birth and death.

For me, every time I think on the "Origins of Everything," I feel bathed by a sense of calm. It's not that my Intellectual Mind is convinced of any facts or that my Survival Mind is clinging to anything tangible. Rather, my Heart-centered Intuitive Mind feels recognized and deeply integrated into the world around me. I feel a sense of oneness with the Universe itself. At times, this feeling comes as a momentary flash. At other times, its sensation sustains and stretches into a lasting inner smile. Surrendering to the unknowable actually weaves us into the radiance of Infinite Consciousness, into the resonance of the One we refer to in many way, as God, as Creator, as life force itself.

It did not matter with whom I studied, a Taoist shaman, the Hawaiian Kahunas, theoretical physicists, Qigong Masters, Christian mystics, Hindu gurus, or Aboriginal elders. The essence of the message was always the same: We live in an amazing Universe gifted to us by a "Creator" and infused with life-force Qi energy. Each one of us is invited to embrace a relationship with this, and it is a deeply individual and personal choice about how we perceive that which lies behind all that is. I trust that by simply engaging in this exploration, it can change our life in amazing ways. In that spirit, enjoy my following personal offering to add to the plethora of creation myths that help us open our mind and Heart to possibilities and ways to question reality:

Teatime with Madam Wuji

One afternoon, you are invited to tea. You sit down, and seated across from you is the infinite and elegant Wuji. She tells you her tale.

For eons, Wuji recounts, she has remained at peace in one eternal experience. The world has lain still in an infinite and primordial field of emptiness. All is silent and still. Suddenly, Hundun appears within the field. Wuji (yin) becomes aware that creation can only exist if she accepts Hundun (yang). Creation is an inevitable part of this dimension, and so Wuji knows she must accept him. Knowing all this, Wuji can still only see

Hundun as darkness, disruptive, and disparaging. He walks with an erratic, disorganized and even violent turbulence that changes what she has always felt was a perfectly fine, calm emptiness. She peers out and watches as Hundun wreaks havoc across the Universe. She wonders, is this tumultuous darkness to be the way of unfolding now and forevermore? She lies still, continuing to observe the endless assault taking place in every corner of her once peaceful emptiness. Darkness prevails and her despair continues. She concludes that this is how life will be from now on.

Just as quickly as she can make her conclusion about the way that Hundun will walk this dimension forever, a glimpse expresses itself to her that feels different. For a moment, there is a brightness far off in the distance, an incredible brightness that she had never experienced before. All she had ever known of "light" was the way it was defined by Hundun's darkness. Drawn to this brightness, she fought despair with all her might so that she could move and travel over to it. There at its source she found a star. A glowing, warm, vibrant sun emerged out of her emptiness. In all her time being Wuji, she had never seen anything like this in her vastness. In fact, she had never seen anything at all, for that is the nature of emptiness. This first "thing" she experienced was beyond description and so she halted every attempt to describe it in order to simply feel the warm, incredible sense of life-force Qi expressing through this brilliant creation. She thought of Hundun and began to feel that maybe he wasn't as bad and destructive as she had imagined. She murmured, "if his presence could bring such a brightness into existence, maybe what was my despair was really just resistance. Perhaps the darkness was that I had never known lightness."

In that moment, Hundun emerged from behind the star smiling upon Wuji. She smiled back, though still wary. Hundun said, "I understand what all this may have seemed like. I didn't know how to describe brightness to you when you had no reference. By you seeing the darkness in me, I knew that you would then understand the creation of light itself." Wuji now saw Hundun as neither dark nor light, but simply the force critical for creation in all its forms. From that moment on, Wuji and Hundun danced together for eons as more and more stars came into being. As the Universe filled with light, Wuji continued to embrace infinite potential while Hundun drew out the alchemical tapestry, with the help of Qi, to bring brilliance to every corner of the Universe.

Meet the Qi Effect

Before we get into the Qi Effect itself, it is important to first look at a specific belief system that has existed since the dawn of humanity. It will be difficult to go further until we look at a simple, self-defining world view, one that you will now need to make a personal choice about, in order to move further:

Conduit vs Container

For decades, I've posed these two contrasting models and views we hold about ourselves to many people around the world in my workshops and lectures. I've watched some people debate the idea in a struggle to justify their disempowering beliefs while others receive that "metanoia" intuitive flash when their minds change gears and they see a new way of being. Sometimes the simplest ideas are the most profound.

I pose this core question about our conditioned belief: "Are we physical/material beings in a physical/material world, or are we energetic beings in a world of energy?" This question points to everything we explored in the last chapter and defines the massive shift to materialism over the past 500 years after millennia of naturally embracing a world of spirit and energy.

Around one hundred years ago, many great scientific minds made the amazing shift to look at the world around us in terms of "energy quanta." This opened science to accept on solid mathematical terms what was termed Quantum Physics. You have to appreciate that this was 100 years ago, and that science is still trying to resolve many of the questions that arise from these concepts. In 1905, Albert Einstein who actually had a hard time accepting Quantum Physics, showed mathematically that not only is there a direct relationship between the material world and energy, but that they are in fact interchangeable. This is how the atomic energy came into being that humans use in a wide spectrum of applications from weapons to the massive generators that power the grid. The scientific community had to undergo a paradigm shift before being able to apply this concept practically and build numerous and commonplace useful devices.

"The Equivalence of Mass and Energy," is a 2001 article in the Stanford Encyclopedia of Philosophy. It reads, "In relativistic physics, as in classical physics, mass and energy are both regarded as properties of physical systems or properties of the constituents of physical systems. If one wishes to talk about the physical stuff that is the bearer of such properties, then one typically talks about either 'matter' or 'fields.' The distinction between 'matter' and 'fields' in modern physics is itself rather subtle in no small part because of the equivalence of mass and energy. Philosophically, to think of fields as stuff is also controversial. Nevertheless, we can assert that whatever sense of 'conversion' seems compelling between mass and energy, it will have to be a 'conversion' between mass and energy, and not between matter and energy."

You may want to read that again and let it sink in. The article illuminates how the scientific community is clinging to the materialistic description of the physical world as "matter." They can still say that "mass" and "energy" are interchangeable, hence Einstein's Equation and General Theory of Relativity, but allowing the world of "matter," things we see and feel, to have equivalence with energy appears too hard to accept.

Arthur Eddington, the famous English physicist and astronomer, stated in 1929 that "it seems very probable that mass and energy are two ways of measuring what is essentially the same thing." This is the commonly accepted viewpoint in science today. Notice the deliberate choice of the word "mass" and not "matter."

Over 100 years has unfolded since these amazing breakthroughs dislodged us from Newtonian materialism, but the full release into accepting that the world around us can in fact be better described as an energetic field effect still has not occurred. This stubborn separation of the material world from the world of energy blocks us from discussing the Qi Effect in the energetic world view.

What we can do is discuss a question that has a real and dynamic impact on how you view your life. This returns us back to the belief system we started the chapter off with. The idea here is that we typically see ourselves in one of two diametrically different ways, either as a Conduit or as a Container.

If we choose the Container perspective, this self-view fits perfectly into the conditioning that we explored earlier. That conditioned view that thriving meant getting more and more into your "container" has become the modern measure of success. When we see ourselves as a Container, we operate from the limits that define the container. It's borders will dictate its dimensions and volume, its structural integrity, and so forth. This, in many ways, describes the Newtonian world view of closed-loop, finite systems. If you are the type that operates your life from this Container perspective, you will naturally be concerned with filling your container, being careful not to drain your container, protecting your container, and generally thinking about how other people view the way you handle your Container duties and how your box-like Container looks. Your Container can be understand as your physical body, the way your think, and/or your self-identity.

Containers "box" us in.

As it relates to Qi, maintaining a Container belief system will keep you busy collecting Qi to fill your Container. It will keep you busy watching for leaks in fear that you might lose Qi. You will notice how you spend an inordinate amount of time and energy protecting and defending your energy. All the while, you will be consumed with the fear, anxiety, and worry of managing your precious Container. Sadly, this way of thinking is in alignment with how most people have been taught to practice Qigong. Holding to this perspective and belief system will both influence the view you convey to the world around you and influence the world that mirrors that view.

If we instead choose the Conduit perspective, we choose the path of courage and Trust. To be a Conduit, you must release your need to contain and protect anything. This includes Qi. It requires the unconditional trust of your Intuitive Mind. A Conduit is a channel. In this world view, you are being asked to trust your immersion in Qi energy and resist the urge to "store" it. You are asked to feel from your deepest place of knowing that Qi, life force energy, is infinitely present everywhere… and exists infinite supply. This means that you have to Trust that energy will be there when you need it without allowing fear to drive you to hold or store it. While the Container has a belief that there is a finite volume of Qi to work with, the Conduit has the ability to tap into the infinite field of Qi. As a Conduit, there is nothing to "protect." Rather, you are a channel immersed in the infinite. As a Conduit, your view of what others may think is irrelevant since you are channeling Qi Activation in and out and through. As such, you are completely immersed in the world around you. In this immersion, the idea of separation inherent in the Container view dissolves away and is transformed into a fully entangled energy connection. A Conduit is integrated into and is at one with the Universe itself including others all around you. This takes massive Trust and sensitivity to release one's isolated Ego identity and still feel safe. This takes a Heart-centered world view and lifestyle.

Living a lifetime as a Container, you've most likely built an identity in order to manage that Container and provide you a certain level of security, albeit a false, illusory security. That self image you've held most of your adult life has dictated your career choices, your self esteem, your relationships, your family interactions, and yes, even your health.

Sure, being conscious of the times we choose "Container" is part of what it means to live consciously Awake in this world. We do live in a world dominated by Containers and Container Mentality. Choosing our identities and making them work for us consciously is a life skill. Allowing our identities to control us and force us to make life choices in ways that sustain the Container limitations is what leads to frustration and illness as it drains us on the deepest level. An isolated Container is disengaged from fully activating Qi in effortless and efficient ways. Feel into that one, it's so important.

Back in the mid '70s, my first Master teacher had a rich background studying both in China and in Japanese Zen monasteries. As a young man, he personally practiced with Carl Jung and Sigmund Freud in Austria and France. What I found to be even more influential, to him and as a result to me, was that he studied in Paris with G.I. Gurdjieff. Gurdjieff was the Russian mystic who created the 4th Way School, melding many empowering concepts from different schools of ancient thought. He believed that most people lived their life in a "waking sleep," which heavily influenced him to focus on releasing the identities (Containers?) we are unknowingly trapped in. Gurdjieff was a Master of many things beyond spiritual studies including cooking, dance choreography, writing, music, and martial arts. He was the ultimate "Conduit," in that he seemed to channel whatever was required in the moment in a way that gave him mystical qualities. Of the many stories my teacher shared with me about the times he spent with Gurdjieff, one that stuck with me was when my teacher was studying under Gurdjieff. My teacher, along with his fellow students, hadn't heard from him in weeks and had been left wondering what had happened. One day while walking in the public market, they heard a hawker selling carpets so loudly that it drew their attention. To their amazement, the "hawker" was Gurdjieff himself. He went on ranting to the passing crowd about the quality of the carpet in his hand. Without missing a beat, he turned from a prospective sale to his young students and said sternly, "Where have you been? Class is tomorrow in the meeting room off the Champs-Élysées." He then went back to selling carpets. He consciously embodied whatever identity he chose at whatever appropriate time, changing from one to the other at will. He "owned" the Container he chose to use when the moment required, consciously used it, and consciously released it. He was Awake from his subconscious Sleep, truly a free spirit. I noticed this characteristic in every one of the authentic and effective Master teachers I studied with to one extent or another.

For some of us, making the conscious choice between Conduit and Container is not that easy… we have a lifetime of conditioning to undo. We may have spent our entire lives working tirelessly to maintain our Container only to find that it left us drained, never giving us the time we thought we would have to savor true satisfaction. This typically happens during times of career change, the end of a relationship, an illness, or a mid-life crisis. During these times of tumult, we simply arrive at the inner knowing of our Intuitive Mind that our Container no longer serves us. A side or two fall from the Container molded so completely to as we open up into the Conduit. Perhaps we hear the wisdom of the Intuitive Mind that this Conduit nature is the only way we can truly go on living.

A dear friend of mine took Qigong workshops from me for several years while he worked in the provincial court system for 10 long, hard years. He did what he thought was right even with the struggles that come with being in a career that doesn't match your spirit. He endured as he won the favor of his parents and family for being a good worker. Of course his co-workers and other upwardly mobile friends cheered him on: misery loves company as they say. His beautiful wife, also a dear friend, Yoga instructor, and Qigong student, was in the corporate world and in the midst of Container-land herself. She was happy her husband had a good job even though she wished it was one that didn't leave him so frustrated. With so much societal and peer support, breaking out of a Container-mentality or even seeing it as such is quite a challenge. What is so wonderful about this story is that despite all that, both of my friends made the choice to embrace Conduit consciousness. His wife made the step to trust teaching Yoga full-time. They took their studying and practicing Qigong to Heart and attended workshops together. I watched my friend in workshops and instructor trainings, and over the years I saw his courage blossom. His amazing Heart and Intuitive Mind was given more and more of a chance to influence his life and well-being. His Survival Mind and Intellectual Mind were losing their Container-like grip. Young and in his 30s, he noticed health issues arising from the inner conflict that was at play from not being in full harmony with his Heart, as he was torn trying to maintain his courtroom career. We know now more and more from research that our health is directly related to stress. When stress increases, our cortisol levels rise in our bloodstream and our immune system becomes highly compromised. He followed his Heart and got Certified to be a Qigong Instructor in one of the courses I offer, and he made the leap into his Conduit nature. With his courage clear and present, and with the loving support of his wife, friends, and even one of his coworkers, he quit his career. Only from being Heart-centered and tapping into that Intuitive Mind energy can we adopt a Conduit way of being. My friend's life and health has changed dramatically for the better. I love this couple and they are the model relationship to me because of their mutual support, trust, and true friendship.

For some people, it is absolutely overwhelming to think about being a Conduit and thus, they choose the illusory safety of a Container. They may also not trust that there will be enough Qi energy, or other resources for that matter, available at the time they need it if they adopt Conduit consciousness. They thus opt for the Container world view so that they can at least cling to the belief that they have some Qi they've stored up, even if it is very limited and frustrating most of the time. How easily we get conditioned to endure disempowering belief systems... How long does it take before we love ourself enough to break out of the Container that cages us?

You probably can see yourself as either a Conduit or a Container, right? Maybe there are some places in your life where you are a Conduit while in other circumstances you are a Container. This is normal human behavior, but I venture to guess that most of our human behavior is subconsciously driven and creates the generally insane world that we see around us.

Bouncing back and forth between Conduit and Container perspectives is one of the most stress-related and emotionally draining challenges we experience in life. Think about it for yourself even if you haven't described it that way before. Think about the circumstances where you are absolutely in your joy, where you are in a trusting space. Being a Conduit is effortless. These are usually situations where you are in your comfort zone and where you feel safe. Your experience tells you that you can succeed in a task, trust a person or situation, or just let go and relax. We all know these moments, whether it be at work doing a job we are good at and get praise for, or when we are doing something we love, like playing music or enjoying walking on the beach during a vacation. You feel that you are "in the zone" and tapped into to the Universe. Everything is flowing smoothly, and you embody the Conduit.

Then there are those "other" times when everything is a struggle and even your efforts seem useless. Emotions run high and you feel trapped. Maybe you even feel like a victim. These are some of the signs that Container mode has set in. Typically when fear takes hold, we opt for the Container world view. It's usually not even a conscious choice, but a reactionary coping mechanism that comes from our Survival Mind triggered by our "old brain" and amygdala. Think about the sympathetic nervous system "fight or flight" response we are familiar with. It is these subconscious and many times epigenetic influences that keep us shackled to old, chronic, disempowering patterns. This is why learning about activating Qi through a specific and empowering Qigong practice can be just the "sensitivity training" we need to transform the subtle drivers that keep us in fear mode and make it so difficult to be free. Qigong practice builds interoception, or body awareness, and this sensitivity begins to extend to energetic sensitivity. Much research on this such as Interoception: A Multi-Sensory Foundation of Participation in Daily Life by Carolyn M. Schmitt and Sarah Schoen show the critical value of somatic (body) awareness and "the interplay between the brain and the body that necessary to maintain homeostasis (good health) as well as respond adaptively to the changes in one's internal and external environment." With this physical and energetic sensitivity, we gain trust through personal, first-hand experience, and watch the territorial limits of the Container world view transform into the expansive and freeing Conduit world view.

The stage is now set to explore the Qi Effect. It has been important to explore and understand the concepts of Conduit and Container so that we may see how they relate to our self view. Our self view is the belief system that we carry about our identity. Even if you have accepted that much of your life experience is in the Container mode, don't worry... join the club. What is key, as Gurdjieff pushes for, is that we wake from our Sleep and wake up from solely being controlled by our subconscious drives and conditioning. Just knowing about this influence will put you in a completely different category than most people on this planet. I call it becoming part of the CommunityAwake. No one is perfect or perfectly Awake. Our motivation should be to stay as Awake to our subconscious drives as much as possible for as much of the time as possible. In this way, they have less and less chance to get the better of you. Stay vigilant, observe, and release self-judgement... simply watch and make choices to embrace your Conduit nature. What did St. Francis of Assisi say? "All the darkness in the world cannot extinguish the light of a single candle." Staying Awake with a Heart-centered consciousness is your candle... and all your subconscious manipulation is simply the darkness...

Knowing that your true nature is not your Container-like identity is critical, and is a game-changing step for each of us towards freedom. On top of it all, there is another very important belief system shift that must be adopted, or at least invited in, in order to really embrace the Qi Effect.

If Qi is life-force energy then the question arises, does it affects my physical body or just my energy body?

This is a good question, and one that points directly to a few more questions that we need to get clear about before we go further. Are we physical bodies with a slight energetic component? Are we energy/

spirit with an apparent physical component? Or are we just energy and everything else is illusion?

Of course, these are the questions that have challenged the best minds in history. From religions to research labs, these questions lie at the very core of our belief system. These socially-accepted authorities actually force us to accept an answer so that we can move forward as a collective. We either embrace and explore challenging new theories and concepts about our energetic nature or simply accept that we are just physical, biological lifeforms that struggle to survive. The latter never sits well and has spawned ardent scientists who struggle to make some sense of it all… and where they fail, religion usually takes over. This book is definitely not my forum to give any answers on the religious side. I celebrate all spiritual beliefs and support each person to listen to their Heart and their religious/spiritual guides. These are deeply personal matters and define us at the core, and that's beautiful.

My intention in writing this book is to look at the three italicized "are we" questions above and come to some consensus about the bio-energetic nature of who we are. When we can do this, the Qi Effect will make a lot more sense and become a practical tool for our health, well-being, and personal life transformation.

To answer these fundamental questions about the nature of the world we live in let's look at something pretty much know and accept: that we are made up of atoms. This includes our bodies and everything we see around us. Of course "atom" is a Greek word like so many of our words in English and Latin-based, Romance languages. Originating in the 5th Century BCE, atom means "uncuttable" because it was believed to be the most fundamental, unbreakable building block. The pre-Socratic minds who evolved our vocabulary were amazing and intuited that there was something primary at the very core of our physical structure. The Methodic School, a medical philosophy in ancient Greece, held a theory that it was the disruption of the normal circulation of "atoms" through the body's "pores" that cause disease. This example shows how people intuitively sense that we are made up of something we can't see, and that this "something" needs to move and align in a harmonic state for us to stay healthy.

It is fascinating that it took 2,300 years after the ancient Greeks for the scientific community to once again agree that we are made up of atoms. Then, only 100 years ago, we finally realized that atoms are not even the smallest, "uncuttable" elements of our universe with the discovery of sub-atomic particles. We've all learned in school about electrons, neutrons, and protons: the sub-atomic components that make up atoms. The average person really doesn't care much about this, but this discovery completely turned the scientific community upside down. It all started back in the late 1890's, when physicists from England, New Zealand, Denmark, and Germany started to understand how atoms where constructed. Over the next 20 years, it became clear that the atom was not the smallest building block of the physical world, and that there were smaller, sub-atomic particles that created the atom. This was a big relief, of course, for classical physicists because now they could get their hands on all the tangible new bits and parts (particles) and impose their mathematical calculations on them to show that the human mind can in fact have a total and complete grasp on knowing everything about, and thereby controlling, the physical world. We sorta know were that attitude leads us…

Very soon, the scientific community started falling apart. In 1905 Albert Einstein, the German-turned-Swiss PhD physicist working as a Patent Office clerk, presents his paper to the scientific community on special relativity and mathematically proved the mass-energy equivalence. Although we all know the equation E=mc2, not many of us embrace the clear significance of the fact that matter and energy are absolutely interchangeable. The elegant and safe materialistic model of Classic Physics was completely turned upside-down and Sir Issac Newton probably also turned upside-down in his grave. From a safe and predictable world where energy, time, and matter were clearly defined and were absolutes that could

MEET THE QI EFFECT

be measured, Einstein and his contemporaries catapulted science into a world where they were stretchable and interchangeable.

Within another dozen years, science went through its next tsunami tumult and started to realize that it couldn't even explain why we can't pinpoint an electron's location at any one time if we also knew its momentum. Physicists realized that all we had was a slight probability of knowing anything at all and for heaven's sake, why did those pesky electrons seem to behave as much like a sound wave as they did as a particle? Uncertainty is a wonderfully disconcerting motivator that most of us try to control through coping skills and by clinging to some feel-good belief system lest fear creep in and makes a mess of things. By 1925, Werner Heisenberg, the German theoretical physicist wrote his seminal paper on the "Uncertainty Principle" stating basically that we really can't know all details about anything in any given moment. This was a year after the French physicist Louis de Broglie made the breakthrough discovery that not only electrons, but everything atomic and sub-atomic behaves as much like a wave as it does a particle. With this came the massive evolution in science we know as Quantum Physics. I like remembering that the word "quantum" is simply the Latin word that means "how much" and gives us the word "quantity." The quantity that this new field of science focuses on is the dynamic, energetic field effect of absolutely everything around us that we once considered to be solid matter.

All of that was just 100 years ago. In this past century, we have continued to delve deeper into the sub-atomic world thanks to billion-Euro toys for Quantum Physicists called particle accelerators that smash atoms to pieces for fractions of a second. All of this tells us that even though we have discovered "particles" smaller than electrons, neutrons, and protons called quarks, colors, and other exotic participants, we really still don't know much about the inner workings of the atom. What remains quite clear and accepted is that everything is based on a "quanta" of energy. This is where the term Quantum Physics comes from. Everything is still made of atoms (thank heavens for the Greeks) but the atom is actually a field of energy, a resonant quantum field. The coherence of this field is the amalgam of the atomic orbital effect. This is the energetic pattern created by the probabilities of the electron "cloud" and the amazing patterns that they create called "atomic orbitals."

You should read about this yourself so that you don't think I'm on some New Age tangent. This is pure science in the 21st Century! Trust me, it is a challenge for scientists as well, whether they work in the area of physics or biology. Everything is a dancing field of energy.

When I was a child, I envisioned each of us as being an energy field. I was surprised when I soon discovered that other people actually didn't feel this at all, just like they didn't have the "starfield dreams" I was having either. This was a curious awakening that helped me wake up to the vastly different realities each of us have. It's probably also what propelled me into my regular meditation practice. I was 7 or 8, and can this remember because we had just moved into a new house. The new environment triggered new things in me; my meditations happened spontaneously at first. I was lying on my bed and the fingers of my hands met at my belly area. Fingertips of one hand met fingertips of the other... then there was a little adjustment and just way a key enters a lock, something shifted. I'm not the type to get scared or let questions block my flow, so I went with what was occurring and it was lovely. The point of view of my awareness was no longer me laying on my back but was from the ceiling down. I can recall this now, 55 years later, as if it was happening now. Maybe it's because it was so natural and pleasant. I remember that the more I used my fingertips to guide my meditations, the more comfortable I was with "traveling" my awareness outside of the room, above the house, over the yard, and nearby areas like the park, the forest, and the river. Something told me not to go too far and I was ok with that. Something told me that these experiences were to help me see things for what they were. Even though we have bodies and the world appears physical, we can easily transcend those limits even if just for a moment, and remember how much more there is to this experience of life...

If atomic orbitals are actually windows into the coherent energy fields that make up the signature of each atom in the Periodic Chart, then they carry a certain type of information and intelligence. This would mean that each atom carries a quantum of information in its energetic matrix. This "intelligence" may not seem the same as what we think of when we use our Intellectual Minds, but at some level it is. The word "intelligence" comes from the compound Latin "intelligere" made up of the words "inter" (between) and "legere" (to read). Intelligence may then be defined as "to be able to read from all the information present." An atom is therefore intelligence incarnate, as each atom carries a unique matrix of information that stays coherent and consistent through its unique subatomic constituents. This is why science can predict some things with certainty and why physicists and engineers can rely on the material world, for the most part, to consistently behave as they would like.

Now if we accept that each atom is a quantum of intelligence, and that each atom is essentially a wave function of an energetic field, then our physical world is a massively complex network of intelligent, energetic wave resonances. Yes it is solid, and tangible, physical, and many times very expensive and annoying. But this is because at our gross level of granularity, our "normal" perspective of things are of things. It's what happens when we give in idea of the world being made of stuff to deal with. There is something called the "weak force" within each atom that basically holds the sub-atomic elements together. It is actually far stronger than gravity, creating the incredible density of atoms that allows our world to appear solid. The "weak force" makes it easier to drive your car or brush your teeth. Yet at the essential level, beyond the trap of looking at things one way from a physical perspective, the world around us is a fabulous dance of energy camouflaged as the things you see. It is only our limited perspective of the five senses that traps us in limitation.

It is at this point that we have to return to Qi. We now have the bridge of contextual framework for how this life-force energy may fit in and become a significant game-changer in our life and health.

I can imagine what you may be thinking, we just talked about all those amazing European scientists who cracked the code to the atomic structure and on a silver platter delivered us a plethora of equations defining every single aspect of physical and energetic interaction. So why didn't they mention Qi? And why, in the ensuing 100 years since Quantum Physics first broke open a new, more complete but not yet unified view of reality, haven't we seen the mention of Qi?

Until we can answer these questions, the Qi Effect won't make any sense. Nor will it fit neatly into the mix, although I think you will soon see how it does. If we want to get to the bottom of our queries, these days the only avenue inside the world of sub-atomic particle research is to visit a physicist and a particle accelerator. Before we can even take an experiment to a particle accelerator, we must first become a physicist. After that, we must spend months if not years making calculations. We must then compile our calculations into a very precise protocol for an experiment. Only then can we apply to the facility review board, and wait sometimes years, to get an hour, if we're both fortunate and well funded, to run the experiment at someplace like the CERN Large Hadron Collider (LHC) particle accelerator near Geneva, Switzerland. This 27-kilometer (over 16 miles) long device uses high-power magnets to accelerate atoms so that they can collide with each other at speeds approaching the speed of light. Why do we spends millions of dollars doing these experiments? So that particle physicists can explore the sub-atomic particles that are emitted from atoms in these high-speed collisions. The massive energy created by these collisions shows up on the LHC detectors just like a picture appears on a TV screen, proving that subatomic particle emission occurs. Seeing this gives us tangible proof that the sub-atomic particles that are the building blocks of atoms actually exist! And that is a good thing for the scientific mind. The challenge is that it also creates exotic new atomic structures that only last a fraction of a second and defy the logic of what we though was possible. Many of those subatomic particles seem to disappear and leave this dimension while others appear and enter it, just as we discussed in the last chapter relating to String Theory and "degrees of freedom."

I know this can all sound unrelated, but trust me, it leads us back to the Qi Effect in a most curious way.

If we agree that we are immersed in an infinitely vast field of life-force, life-giving energy we call Qi, then it begs the question, "Where is it." All my lovely New Age friends and energy healers tend to agree with Traditional Chinese Medicine, Classical Chinese Medicine, Qigong, and Reiki practitioners. They say that Qi is all around us. Many say that they can "feel the Qi" flowing through the body. What's most curious is that not a single person can show evidence of its presence in this dimension. No one can show it under a microscope or measure it on any meter. I personally spent years living in China building trust with researchers and scientists interested in these matters. In the documentary that I produced and directed on Qigong back in 1999, I interviewed several researchers doing their best to measure Qi. Many were well-funded scientists and had government support, yet they couldn't conclusively say they were measuring "Qi." They all used various measurement devices for electromagnetic waves, making field function measurements ranging from heat to sound to light. Although they measured many energy bandwidth changes, it was clear that these were not Qi. The changes in energy bandwidth showed the "effect" of Qi. Although this is a subtle point, it is a critical one. If you are actually measuring heat, sound, light or other electromagnetic waves, you are not measuring Qi. You are measuring the Qi Effect, the way Qi expresses in our world. I believe what those scientists were measuring is exactly what we experience when we practice Qigong. It isn't Qi itself, but in fact it is the Qi Effect. To say you "feel" Qi or are "measuring" Qi creates the problem I see in many energy healers who shift their focus away from fully activating the Qi Effect, and limit their sensory perspective only to aspects of the physical world. It's a bit like saying you had a private dinner with movie star when you really only watched them in a video stream while you were eating at home. You would question the person's sanity if they tried to convince you that they actually shared that meal in an intimate way, just as I question people saying that they are "feeling Qi." Saying that you feel Qi cheats you out of truly experiencing what is occurring when your body and energy transform through the way you are "activating" Qi. This brings us into a more authentic relationship with life-force energy; Qi isn't forced it into the space/time limits of this dimension and a newly expansive, sensory experience unfolds in the process. When trap ourselves by experiencing life only through our senses, which are incredibly limited and bound within this dimension, we literally lock ourselves out of the massive possibilities available when we expand our perception into other dimensions, such as the one where Qi resides. When we understand that our practice, whatever it may be, is actually all about activating the relationship between Qi and our physical/energetic realm, our healing and transformational experience will be greatly enhanced.

The Qi Effect is simply how Qi influences and affects our body, energy field, and everything around us.

Every year, it becomes more and more clear that Qi is not of this dimension even though it works through this dimension at the subatomic level. My increasing experience and clarity on these matters has brought me a growing sense of inner peace. Let us take everything that we have learned from Quantum Physics and the energy-mass equivalence, and combine it with our own spiritual intuition and the many teachings of ancient wisdom. All of it seems to point out that the world that surrounds us is as much a dynamically shifting energetic field as it is a physical one, and that they merge and meld in absolutely natural ways. We all have had experiences where we watched spontaneous healing within ourselves and others. We have all had experiences of synchronicities such as "knowing" who was on the other end of the phone before we looked down to see who was calling. Many of us have had intuitive moments that defy the logical limits of a material world constrained by the speed of light.

These seemingly amazing experiences of instantaneous synchronicity are windows into the Qi Effect: they are the very real effect of Qi interfacing with our dimension. When the Qi Effect occurs, it appears to shift the rules and limitations of space/time that our five senses have trapped us in. This is exactly what we described in the last chapter when we discussed stars and molecular clouds forming in the depths of apparently "empty" space. Science is baffled by this, and created the term "dark matter" to try and explain how in the "empty" space where stars form, mass can exist that can't be seen. The "dark" mass that we can't "see" that exists within the "empty" space where stars form exists even before the stars begin to farm. The phrase "dark matter"appears exotic, but astrophysicists call it "dark" because they just don't know what it is. Since "dark matter" has measurable mass, I can logically deduce that it is the subatomic transitory-state of "energy-becoming-matter," similar to what happens inside star-forming hydrogen clouds. We are in a Universe where energy and mass are woven together, and though Einstein and others made that clear, the limited scientific mind can't accept the life-force Qi Effect until it is tangible and measurable. There is a natural "creation" process taking place every second of every day throughout the Universe that has gone on forever, and will continue indefinitely.

Every atom in every molecule of every cell in our body is a micro-expression of these star fields. How can they not be? They carry their quantum memory from their origin, which began inside of a star. At the level of quarks, every subatomic particle appears to be moving in and out of this physical realm. In various degrees of freedom, these particles move out of this "dimension" and return to their atomic quantum field coherence. This continual state of transitory flux sustains homeostatic harmony. It all happens in tiny fractions of a second, so the world appears stable to our limited sensory perspective. Nonetheless, it is happening all of the time. Could this be how Qi plays its role? Though Qi may not be physically present in this dimension, the subatomic elements (which we know are really coherent vibrating quantum fields) have the ability to pass into the dimension of Qi and return to our physical realm "recharged." This weaving interrelationship of energy and matter is actually totally consistent with Einstein's Equation, and all of the subsequent refinements and special cases posed by physicists in the ensuing 100+ years.

Remember that everything with mass can also be described in energetic terms. Electromagnetic fields are by nature energetic and every aspect of our body emits an electromagnetic field. This means that the field around our body, named the Wei Qi field by the ancient Taoists, is simply an electromagnetic field and not actually Qi. The fractional frequencies of this electromagnetic field would also have the natural ability to move in an out of this dimension in order to be recharged by the Qi Field in its dimension. This is in part how we feel the Qi Effect in our practice or healing.

This concept may intuitively feel absolutely "right" to you. Wonderful. This may sound like something far-fetched and sci-fi. Also wonderful. These ideas may seem "wrong" because they don't fit into what you've studied about Qigong, Yoga, or energy practice so far. Still wonderful. That you've stayed with the book this long means that you know in your Intuitive Mind that what you've been told in your life up to now has not been the whole story.

Biologists study something called "magneto reception" when they attempt to understand how bats, dolphins, migratory birds, pigeons, and turtles determine their spatial location, heading direction and navigational goal endpoint that is sometimes thousands of miles away. Even the biologists, who study the specific brain activity of these beautiful animals to see which regions of their neural networks fire during various phases of navigation, don't understand the full workings of the process. We realize that these creatures are far more advanced than humans in sensing the electromagnetic fields that surround themselves and the Earth. Yes, it is the energy fields that are all around us that they not only sense, but can read in fine detail. Comparatively, humans walk around blind and unaware of this amazing field of information radiating everywhere on the planet. Without a smartphone and its satellite-dependent GPS, the average human wouldn't be able to drive to the next town. Yet a wide array of those in the animal community live with a consciousness of the relationship between their Wei Qi field and the Earth's. I'd go as far as to say that most all animals, including many insects (think of the Monarch Butterfly that migrates over

2,000 miles each season) are sensitized and conscious to the ever-present electromagnetic fields.

We know that our planet, like all others, carries an electromagnetic field that surrounds it in the shape of a torus. It projects from the South Pole as a positive electric charge, travels up past the equator where it becomes somewhat neutral, and then returns to enter the North Pole as a negative charge. This is basic geologic science. What's curious is that you may not realize that this electromagnetic charge has a measurable signature, charge value and angle at any and all points on Earth. The Earth radiates that signature for those adept to recognize it, and a sensitive creature would be able to tell their exact longitude and latitude on the planet at any time. We see this from the way turtles return to the exact same location to lay eggs after being far at sea for months. We see it in the way a pigeon can fly miles and miles and return to a tiny cage. This is the depth of what quantum physicists refer to as the wave function: the precise energetic character and possibilities inherent in our field of existence. Yes, humans have a lot to "remember" about what we know on a cellular level, yet it has been bred out of us as we developed our Intellectual Mind. This actually took place over tens of thousands of years through what is known as "evolutionary genetics." Over the process of evolution, various genes whose tasks were no longer required, either got "turned off" or actually dropped from our DNA. Although genes literally carry the intelligence to manufacture all the proteins in our body, that same "intelligence" contributes to our subconscious awareness as well as our conscious thoughts. The takeover of our Intellectual Mind has simultaneously been accelerated through social conditioning and in the last Century, through technology. We have become more and more dependent on myriad technologies to do things for us which has led to a lifestyle migration away from nature and into suburban and urban housing. The skills, conscious or subconscious/genetic, that you don't exercise and keep in practice, you lose. Remember that we share nearly the whole genome with our animal cohabitants on this planet, so it is more about what we have forgotten to utilize as a human species skill set than anything else. The Qi Effect is about helping us tap into our latent abilities, knowing that we live in a Qi-infused world that is much more of an energetic vibration than a material structure. It is about rebuilding our natural sensitivities to electromagnetic signatures all around us and in the process, uncovering our amazing natural abilities that typically lie dormant within us.

Doing our personal practices such as Qigong, Yoga, Tai Chi, Reiki, and other energy work may be more critical now than ever in light of increasing EMF (electromagnetic frequencies) being radiated into the world around us. Did you know that nearly 10,000 active satellites circle overhead in low Earth orbit, all radiating a variety of EMF ranging from radio to 5G cellular emissions and beyond? Did you realize that another 17,270 satellites have already been approved by the U.S. Federal Communications Commission (FCC) to be launched into space soon, with another 65,912 satellite applications pending at the time of this writing? Many of these will be radiating intense 5G EMF to the entire Earth 24 hours per day. Sadly there is not much we can do to stop this madness although countless members of the scientific community have warned of the dangers of this increased EMF to humans, animals, and the Earth's sensitive, toroidal magnetic field. Arthur Firstenberg is just one scientist who states, "Everyone is completely blind to is the effect of all the EMF radiation from satellites on the ionosphere, and consequently on the life force of every living thing. The relationship of electricity to Qi and Prana has escaped the notice of modern humans. Atmospheric physicists and Chinese physicians have yet to share their knowledge with one another. And at this time, such a sharing is crucial to the survival of life on Earth." Our personal energy practice and understanding of the Qi Effect will define who stays healthy in the coming years and who will fall prey to the array of negative health effects that have been proven beyond the shadow of a doubt. Practices like Qigong help to strengthen and ground our personal Wei Qi energy field which helps to counter the toxic effects of EMF. Inquisitive physicists have understood the facts about the energetic component of life for centuries, yet many of them have been pushed into obscurity because it doesn't fit into the mainstream narrative.

Ruggero Giuseppe Boscovich was a physicist you probably never heard of, yet he influenced great scientists such as Michael Faraday, Sir William Hamilton, James Clerk Maxwell and Lord Kelvin, and even the philosophers Nietzsche and Kant. In the 1740s, Boscovich was a mathematician, physicist, and astronomer who wrote more than 70 groundbreaking papers on a variety of subjects and curiously did a fair bit of work with the Vatican. It is very likely that he had access to the vast and secretive Vatican Library and it is believed that much of his advanced concepts came from knowledge that was hidden from the public in documents held secure in that library. His writings critiqued the work of Liebniz and Newton and improved on their theories of physical reality. His concept of a "center of oscillation" was a step towards an energetic description of matter, and this was in conflict with Newton and the Church that supported him. Most likely this is why Boscovich was nudged into obscurity where Newton and his practical materialism was exalted. Things (and bodies) that are of material nature can be quantified and controlled by the powers that be, yet things (and bodies) that are energetic in nature have lots more "degrees of freedom" and can't be controlled. Ultimately, Boscovich couldn't accept that light could be a wave because he couldn't fully break from seeing everything as material. His concept of "puncta" was that there is an energetic and oscillating center point in all materials and objects and that everything exists within an energetic "ether." Seeing that this was nearly 300 years ago, it is amazing that he intuited the energetic component of the material world and shifted the conception of the atom from a rigid "thing" into a vibratory field. His theories and mathematical equations pushed the stellar minds in science, most likely including Einstein and Tesla as we know they both read Boscovich's famous book written in Latin, "Theoria Philosophiae Naturalis."

If the redefinition of the material world along with the interrelationship between matter and energy is a fundamental principle of all life in this Universe, then the Qi Effect too reflects the very nature of existence by operating in an automated, background way. Stars continue to form, trees grow, babies are born, and all life continues to survive quite on its own without conscious intervention. There is one unique aspect of the Qi

Effect though, and embracing that is why you have been drawn this far along in this book: There is a big difference between just "surviving" by allowing the Qi Effect to operate subconsciously, and "thriving" by being a conscious participant in Qi Activation. Understanding how to embrace and understand the Qi Effect teaches us how to thrive.

The main two things to remember about the Qi Effect is that it is always in action and that we have tremendous influence over its efficiency.

While living in Beijing, I was taught many ancient Taoist phrases and poems along the way. Having a fair bit of free time in between studies with the elder Masters, I would take one of the traditional texts and practice writing it in Chinese calligraphy with a brush and ink. I honored the old ways by making my own ink, taking an ink stone and dissolving it in water. It was a process in and of itself to find the right ink consistency. Then after choosing the correct brush, I painted out the characters, following the correct sequence as each stroke was made in precise order and direction with a proper beginning and ending. It is a beautiful, meditative exercise. Each character has a history and tells a story, projecting its essence as a complete concept. It so different than the Western approach of spelling out a word letter by letter. One of my favorite phrases to practice is a simple concept that took me deep into contemplation. In Pin Yin, the Romanized spelling of Chinese characters, it reads as follows: "Yi Tao, Qi Tao."

When we think of the influence we have over the Qi Effect, this old Taoist phrase may be one of the most important reminders. It uses the character "Yi," which is a very old and misunderstood concept. Many people believe that it means "mind" or "thought." From the very beginning, I sensed this was a very superficial translation of the ancient intent. When I first learned it I described it as "creative visualization." That felt closer to the essence of what my old teachers were trying to share. Even two native Mandarin speaking people might repeat a phrase back and forth several times during a philosophical discussion to ensure that what they were sharing was understood. I've witnessed this many, many times with the elders. Many Mandarin words sound the same yet carry different meanings, so words are typically repeated along with the contextual framework to ensure that the proper meaning is imparted correctly.

The story within the character "Yi" took me years to explore. I knew the accepted definitions fell short of what the ancients intended, and I studied the etymology of this character within old writings to find the depth of meaning I was looking for. The essence of "Yi" is "to bring Qi to Mind." When I read this it, was like a flash of inspiration and clarity. In the next chapter, you will see my drive to clarify what we mean when we use the term "Mind." For now, let's simply think of "Mind" as "our conscious awareness and thinking." The idea of "bringing Qi to Mind" is powerful because it means we are consciously invoking Qi to enter the realm of our awareness, riding on the vibratory waves of thought itself. Remember, electromagnetic waves carry mass and energy the same as subatomic elements. They too can receive the Qi Effect in the form of thoughts or intentions as do subatomic particles.

Looking at the phrase "Yi Tao, Qi Tao," we can deconstruct it further with the word we easily recognize, "Tao." "Tao" is the root word of "Taoism" and may originate from the text supposedly handed down by Lao Tzu titled the "Tao te Ching." We can translate this as "the Way" and in this case, we can think of Tao as "a path traveled." The phrase can now suggest, "Where Yi travels, Qi travels." This is big, and one of the keys to the Qi Effect.

Consider that "Yi" itself suggests that you are using your thoughts and intention to activate the Qi Effect in the mental realm. "Traveling" your Yi then clearly indicates directed awareness. This can be an intention, focus, or even love. The phrase shows that with an enriched awareness of Qi resonance, the Qi Effect can "travel." The intention creates a path, and Qi becomes activated as it travels along that path.

To me, this is the guiding spirit of the Qi Effect. It places deep responsibility on us because probably the only thing that we can really have full responsibility for is the thoughts we choose to think. It's a curious thing to consider, but when you think about it, even "thinking about it" is a choice you make. There are many things in life we don't have such "ownership" over. Our thoughts are completely in our domain. The quality of your thoughts, the choice of your thoughts, the way your direct your thoughts and who you direct them too all are up to you. Realizing this should set off a light inside that grounds you and wakes you up to your potential. If every thought influences the Qi Effect, then everything about your body, health, emotions, relationships, and everything else depends upon the thought selection you allow to sustain in your Mind and awareness.

We realize then that the practice of Qigong, which essentially is how we activate Qi through the Qi Effect, is defined by three key components. Yi, breath, and movement. This is the simple truth of Qigong and of developing your relationship with Qi through the Qi Effect.

The Qi Effect is the activation of Qi to influence all energy in this dimension from material to mental.

To me, Yi is first and foremost. Even if you are just learning about Qigong and it's beautiful moves or exploring breathing techniques, understanding the power and influence of your thoughts is key. There are thousands of Qigong styles. Each one will touch on some aspect of Yi, breath, and movement, for that is what defines Qigong practice. Nei Gong is the class of Qigong that is more internal, meditative, and centered around inner-work. Yi naturally plays an important role in Nei Gong. Yet with any Qigong that follows solid, empowering fundamentals, awareness about the thoughts you carry is critical. Learning to "call Qi to Mind" is a wonderful alignment of our typically chaotic mental processing. Using gentle, deep diaphragmatic breathing to activate the Vagus nerve and thus stabilize heart Qi is how the breath is involved in bathing you in the calm of the Qi Effect. Learning slow, specific movements and stretching will always call on Yi to bring your body, mind, and spirit into a calm that some like to call the "Qi State." We can see how each of these three Qi Gong aspects weave together a tapestry that feels comforting like a blanket wrapping all around you.

I've traveled around the world most of my adult life teaching Qigong and meditation, so I'm typically meeting people interested in living a healthy life. I know that exercising and having a conscious diet are important, but still I meet so many people adhering to those two practices who are still not experiencing optimal health. I've always seen that without embracing the Qi Effect principles, people only get a portion of their required nutrition from eating right and that they often drain themselves during their exercise routine. Until we can incorporate Qi Effect concepts into all we do and shift our perspective to a more energetically-based one, we will only be living a fraction of our potential. When we do, we move from just surviving to truly thriving.

My intention for this book isn't to write a book on Qigong practice, I wrote one of those over 20 years ago and there are lots of books like that already out there. My intention is to help you understand the depths of the Qi Effect itself. Understanding what is taking place in every atom in every molecule of every cell in your body will not only deepen your resolve as to why the practice of Qigong has sustained over millennia, but it will feed your Intuitive Mind and help you to trust what you feel at that body-wisdom level of your life. We have become so convinced that we need to seek out medical experts to tell us what's going on inside our own bodies that we have lost sight of the innate shamanic wisdom we carry. I always say that Qigong is "sensitivity training," a lifelong practice of deepening our inner listening and cultivating our skills of interoception so that we can understand what our body is communicating to us at the subtle energy level before we even experience symptoms related to illness. Interoception is a general term that describes the afferent, body-to-brain intercommunication through specific neural, immune, and endocrine pathways. Clinical research describes mindfulness as "the attentional focus necessary and fundamental for gaining interoceptive skills" (Gibson 2019). Qigong goes much deeper than what we think of as "mindfulness," Qigong-focused breathing paired with intentional movements will refine interoceptive abilities. Research shows that that combination leads not only to physiological homeostatic health, but provides insight into harmonizing our emotions. Emotional harmonization is referred to in medical literature as "emotion regulation" (Valim 2019). This is in part why Qigong is such a powerful, preventative health practice. Research shows that regular practice transforms stress and thereby lowers our blood cortisol levels, strengthens our immune system, rejuvenates our organ systems, and heals our body at deep and lasting levels. If a health issue does arise, increased body awareness builds interoceptive sensitivity so that we can learn to "see" the seeds of symptoms at a very early stage when it is easy to heal what may be out of harmony. Refined sensitivity can help us listen to the emotional influencers within that oftentimes lead to illness. Qigong is a transformational practice that provides us with tools and insights that allow us to see the seeds of emotional disharmony, shift the energetic dynamics at the Heart Resonance level, and activate the Qi Effect in ways that heal us in deep and long-lasting ways.

Many thousands saw my YouTube video post when the agenda to fight the pandemic was first pushed onto an unsuspecting world population. Curiously, it was not censored and taken down like so many others who tried to share their insights and medical findings. Maybe it was because I presented very clearly that it is our individual responsibility to take affirmative action and keep up our daily personal exercise practice, like Qigong, Tai Chi, Yoga, and Meditation, to stay positive and not fall prey to the fear pushed on us by the mainstream media. I also reminded everyone to eat healthy and take the proven and tested, safe nutrients like Magnesium Citrate, Zinc, Vitamin C and D3. Add Quercitin, and this simple protocol is validated to keep our life-long, innate immune system strong naturally. This is the best prophylaxis against any pathogen including viruses, and according to massive data bolsters us far more than any failed attempt at a vaccine.

Let's revisit how we started this chapter by returning to the Container and the Conduit. Now that we have explored the inner workings of the Qi Effect, we can more deeply understand why it is so critical to be clear about which of the two self-perspectives you choose to adopt.

Everything that I have attempted to share here about the Qi Effect speaks to the way our quantum coherent field, whether at the subatomic level or in your thought/electromagnetic field, interfaces with Qi through a most curious, natural set of quantum physics principles. Energy quanta, in the form of subatomic elements or any other type of electromagnetic field, pass into the 'dimension' of Qi, become affected by this lifeforce energetic matrix, and then enter back into our dimension recharged. This is all about flow, but not about Qi flowing. Qi doesn't flow, it simply is. It isn't present in this dimension and thus is not bound by it. It is only the aspects of our space/time dimension that move in a way that we call flow. These aspects are the electromagnetic quantum fields dancing around and through us along with the various subatomic vibratory fields we call particles. All this is in a constant dynamic flux where energy is expressed infinitely in space/time. There is no languaging here about "storage" or "limits" or "blocks" or stagnations." Since these terms are only associated with the limited physics of "Containers," they are also, not surprisingly, associated with illness.

I trust that you will draw the conclusion that the energy physics of our body/mind/spirit is much more in line with Conduit principles when were are in our optimal state of being. Choosing the Conduit world view aligns you with a thriving perspective of vibrant health and efficient Qi Effect activation.

Sir Joseph John (JJ) Thomson, the 1906 Nobel Laureate in Physics, discovered the electron and was famous for his work with electromagnetic and plasma flow. Electromagnetic and plasma flow are concepts that are of conduit nature. Thompson regularly referred back to Michael Faraday who, 100 years before him, did groundbreaking work on electron conductivity and electromagnetic lines of force. Thomson, like Faraday, referred to the conduit nature of energy vibration as "tubes of electrostatic inductance." It is clear that in our physical dimension, charged electrons influence activation fields guided in channels (typically wires). Curiously, Thomson's son, George Paget Thomson, also won the Nobel Prize in Physics. He won the award in 1937 for proving the wave-like properties of electrons. Slowly, science is moving away from rigid material and embracing energy waveforms.

Most people think that electrons flow or move down a wire. The common belief is that when you flip a light switch, the electrons flow from the power source to the lightbulb. This actually isn't true. When a current opens by flicking a light switch on the wall, electrons begin oscillating in place. Remember Boscovich and his "oscillating centers"? Same thing. We think in terms of "flow" because we see a causal action flowing from point A, the light switch, to point B, the lightbulb. In fact, the electrons in the copper wires in the wall don't really move down the wire. Rather, when the circuit is open and activated by throwing the switch, they begin to oscillate and an electromagnetic field is created. This field is contained by the wire and insulation enough to ensure that the light glows. This is the same principle that happens in acupuncture, Qigong, and most all energy work and healing. Qi doesn't move down the meridians, Jing Mai, any more than electrons move along a wire. An electromagnetic field can be activated by an acupuncture needle, pressing on an acupressure point, or simply by engaging a healing intention. When that field is activated beyond normal, autonomic functioning, the Qi Effect is engaged and Qi is activated. This means that subatomic vibratory fields tunnel inter-dimensionally to where Qi resides, get energized, and then return. Occurring in a fraction of a second, these fields become optimized by the Qi interaction and return to their intentional vibratory coherence. In other words, they are reset to their optimal levels. When this is sustained and done correctly, healing takes place.

John Henry Poynting was an English physicist who, in 1884, coined what is known as the Poynting Vector. The Poynting Vector represents a field's energy flow intensity which can be measured in watts per square meter. Poynting clearly figured out the propagation direction of any electromagnetic field along with key information about the energetic capacity moving in that direction. He showed that an electromagnetic wave is composed of an electric field and a magnetic field oscillating in relationship to one another. The cross product of the two fields shows that a "conservation of energy" is at work. "Conservation" here points to the channeling of this new, third energy field along the wire. Electromagnetic energy is never "lost," but is transferred, or conserved, from one state to another. For example, your home space heater transforms electricity into heat.

Our bodies are electromagnetic field generators. This is basic biology 101. We know this because we monitor the brain with EEGs (ElectroEncephaloGrams) and we study the heart with ECGs (ElectroCardioGrams). These devices measure electromagnetic activity in our body, and the state of the relationship between the electric and magnetic fields defines our health. What Poynting saw in electric circuits 150 years ago, we have now discovered in our bodies. When we can see our bodies as a conduit for this energy flux, we have taken a big step in understanding our health and vitality. When we can see our bodies at the subatomic level and understand the conduit nature of Qi Activation, we have taken a giant step in embracing our potential as humans and put the Qi Effect into action.

When you can embrace the Conduit nature of your being, the Qi Effect makes more and more sense. This takes courage and trust. It takes seeing how conditioned you have been your whole life to think you were a Container. This is the main reason people feel disempowered and not in their truth. Trust me, there are many people who teach Qigong from the Container perspective and will attempt to project upon you their fear-based limits and misconceptions. They will try and persuade you to "store" Qi and get rid of "excessive" Qi. They will attempt to convince you that your Qi is blocked or stagnant. It's not about judging them, it's only about listening deeply and choosing what is best for you.

The empowered path of Qigong is not about gathering or clearing Qi, but rather it is about activating Qi.

To activate Qi, we simply need to reorient the way we relate to life-force energy. This means we need to adopt our Conduit nature, truly allowing ourselves to be a channel for the flow of our innate quantum electromagnetic field into the Qi field and back. Yes, we can refer to this as "cultivating Qi" but Qi is fine by itself and infinitely present without needing anything from us. It would be more accurate to say that we are "cultivating the Qi Effect."

Listen to what you hear and read, and then test it against the principles of the Qi Effect. See how the disempowering ideas of limits are so pervasively fear-based and how our life conditioning can easily make us fall prey to these beliefs. I've watched people and even well-meaning teachers attempt to "prove" to me that their anthropomorphized views of Qi were true. It never sat well with me to think that the very life-force, life-giving energy that was infinitely abundant in the Universe would fall prey to the characteristics of a fearful human being. Think about it. As we mentioned before about our poor pets, humans are very good at projecting their limitations and issues on everything around them: alive or not. Humans anthropomorphize everything around them by projecting their problems and unresolved emotional states onto their pets, cars, other people, and even inanimate objects. Qi is not of this dimension, and as such, it cannot be bound to the limitations of this space/time dimension. It is precisely that Qi is unbound that the Qi Effect is what it is. We are all blessed to have access to this resource even if we are normally unaware of how it keeps us alive and the world around us as splendid as it is.

That we are actually given the awareness on how to go deeper into the relationship with the Qi Effect is really a miracle. For some of us, we trust our Intuitive Mind, we trust our "gut," and we observe how just by doing our Qigong practice regularly, we see curious healing events take place. We observe what appears to be illogical healing outcomes even when a physician may have said with absolute certainty that this was impossible. Many of us have an innate sense that the world is more than it appears, and because we can't prove it mathematically or scientifically, we are looked askance at by most people in the world who lie trapped in intellect. Fortunately, I know thousands and thousands around the world that are not affected by the family or friends who don't agree with them. What I do see a lot is that when the nay-sayers get sick and their healthcare providers run out of healing options, they come to us for advice as a last resort. What a shame for people to wait so long to discover the truth of healing and the Qi Effect. Better late than never I suppose.

Another class of people are the ones who want to accept the Qi Effect but are deeply entrenched in their Intellectual Mind. These are people that depend on repeatable scientific facts based on peer-reviewed, placebo-controlled, and hopefully double-blind studies. This pulls in a tremendous number of fear-based people (though they'd never admit this) who don't fully trust their Intuitive Mind and need to be convinced beyond a shadow of doubt. I fully understand this type of person and really appreciate them because if you can show them good data, they will be great supporters of ideas that they would have otherwise relegated to the fringes. This is exactly why I chose to accept the position of President of the Qigong Institute back in the late '90s when it was offered to me by the founder, Dr. Kenneth Sancier, Ph.D.

Dr. Sancier was a Senior Scientist at the prestigious Stanford Research Institute (SRI) and had the pedigree of being an absolutely conservative, mainstream scientist who wrote peer-reviewed papers and was well-accepted by his peers. As fate would have it, as Dr. Sancier got older he got more curious about concepts that were challenging the tenants of the mainstream, especially in the area of bioenergetics. He had heard about the concept of Qi and started to dabble in ways to see if it was quantifiable.

He took the path of galvanic skin response using a device from Japan that used the Ryodoraku method of measuring electrodermal resistance. He did this to trace acupuncture meridians, Jing Mai, with the idea that this is where Qi was "flowing." Dr. Sancier, being the scientist he was, got more curious about the Qigong community in Northern California at the time and actually did experiments to test the before and after effects of practicing Qigong. He started a wonderful database to translate the research being done in China, and then began including his own and other research relating to Qi. I had just returned from living and studying Qigong and Classical Chinese Medicine in China and was in the final phase of producing my television documentary for PBS-TV, so I interviewed Dr. Sancier as part of the documentary. We became fast friends. Before I knew it, he had me on the Board of his non-profit Qigong Institute and I became President. I helped to develop a little CD-based research database into a fully accessible online offering. It became apparent that there was tremendous ongoing research being done around the world in this area that people needed to know about. Through a wonderful set of circumstances, I met a Qigong practicing Silicon Valley engineer named Tom Rogers and brought him onto the Qigong Institute Board. With Tom's tech acumen, we kept expanding the Qigong Database at a rapid rate so that when Dr. Sancier passed from his body in 2013 at the sweet age of 93 years old, Tom's hard work had brought the Database to over 17,000 entries. Dr. Sancier would be pleased to know that we have since expanded the Database to be called the Qigong and Energy Medicine Database which is still a free, online, keyword-based service.

I remain the Chairman of this non-profit, all-volunteer organization because I know the value of research and science to help support those of us who benefit from data to support what we know instinctively. This data comes from renown researchers in universities and medical facilities around the world and is many times listed in the reputable PubMed database. It's legitimacy also helps open the minds of the medical establishment. This is critical in order to return our healthcare system to one based on self-responsibility through lifestyle choices and whole-person healing, and away from pharmaceutical manipulation and disempowerment.

To return to the "science" of the Qi Effect, if you really want to go there and are brave enough to explore the absolute cutting edge of science, you will need to learn about what is being researched not only in Quantum physics, but in Quantum biology. This is where the ride really gets interesting and fully supports my theories on the Qi Effect.

To begin, we must first remember that quantum physics is already over 100 years old. Just because it's not taught in high school as it should be doesn't mean it's pseudo-science in any way. It means that even the basics of quantum physics is beyond the pay scale of most teachers dealing with a classroom full of teens. Quantum physics also introduces two extreme concepts into mainstream thought that don't fit neatly into a world run by corporations and governments that would like people to be well-behaved followers who do as they are told. Why do I say that? Well, because quantum physics states very clearly that the Universe itself is not at all well-behaved and rarely does what it's told! On the other hand, Newtonian rules regarding the physical and material world are exactly what governments, religions, and corporations need to assert their control over the masses. This is why Newtonian constructs and limits have been sustained by "the system" for hundreds of years. It's also why you have heard of Issac Newton and not Ruggero Boscovich. Newton presented a clean view of rigid, materialist atoms while Boscovich presented a world of dancing atoms that oscillate freely. This is no different than why Confucianism supplanted Taoism in ancient China as the power-broker's philosophical tool for mass-conditioning. Confucianism is all about a very specific set of rules, rituals, and beliefs that everyone in society is to follow at all costs. What government seeking to control the masses wouldn't support that philosophy and use it to its own advantage? On the other hand, Taoism is a philosophy that asks the individual to observe the natural world directly for clues on how to live. Taosim asks you to listen for a Universal intelligence that dances within you to guide the flow of life, and it asks you to embrace that there is a life-force called Qi behind all things that is far greater than any set of fixed laws made by man or government. Doesn't this sounds a lot like the shift from Newtonian physics to Quantum physics?

It makes sense to me that Quantum physics would have a difficult time becoming mainstream since it makes us question the very nature of existence. Sure, most of what Quantum physics describes is at either an extreme microscopic, subatomic level or an extremely macroscopic, astronomic level. It plays an elegant role in science by answering questions and describing phenomenon that could not be answered by Newtonian laws of physics. Don't be fooled into thinking that the discoveries of Quantum physics are not applicable to our daily life. Of course nuclear power plants only came into existence because of the paradigm shift in science that finally allowed physicists to accept the laws of quantum mechanics. That's obvious, but what we don't readily realize is that a large portion of the research done in nanotechnology is only possible because of science's understanding of quantum field fluctuations and how energy shifts take place in ways that are only possible when we understand that our physical world behaves much more like electromagnetic waves and dynamic field effects than it does like a rigid machine.

It was only natural that Erwin Schrödinger, the German-born, Austrian-Irish Nobel Prize-winning physicist, wrote in his 1944 book, "What is Life?" about the direction application of Quantum physics into biology. Schrödinger developed many of the key concepts in quantum theory, including his famous equation describing how to calculate the wave function of any system as it transforms over time. In other words, Schrödinger shifted a materialistic view of the world into an energetic one, showing that there were principles in the world of energy as predictable as those in the world of physical objects. Building this bridge from purely physical systems, like nuclear fission/fusion, into biology was the beginning of what has become known as Quantum Biology. It will be key in transforming how we treat disease and maintain health in the future. The challenge is that it requires a complete overhaul of the current biochemistry-based paradigm that keeps Big Pharma in control of healthcare.

Quantum Biology moves us away from seeing the body solely as a complex of biochemical reactions into viewing our whole body as a coherent, intelligent energy field. As Schrödinger stated, a wave function is dynamic and responsive to influences around it including the observers themselves. He referred to our chromosomes, which are made up of DNA in every cell, as aperiodic crystals. This suggests that they store and radiate frequencies (and information) in dynamically responsive ways throughout the body. Rather than limiting our understanding of the human body to the traditional materialistic view, Quantum Biology is moving us toward seeing our bodies from an energy-based perspective. This is making a quantum leap, and the ongoing research in Quantum Physics completely uproots the conditioning in science that limits human evolution and healing to gross genetic mapping and causal biochemical interactions. It is precisely this constricted and arrogant point of view that has allowed us to bend to the will of the large pharmaceutical corporations. Big Pharma has only been able to dominate healthcare because people have allowed themselves to shift from trusting their own body's innate ability to heal and instead are looking outside themselves for a faster and better solution. Once a person buys into that shift, they become more and more susceptible to the incessant pharmaceutical advertising, which is now the dominant revenue source for mainstream media outlets. Our only real path out of this trap comes from the continued discovery that everything is in fact energy: from our bodies to our minds themselves. Quantum Biology actually merges science with what Qigong and energy healing practitioners already know about the powerful body-mind relationship. One of the things that has been "bred" out of humans is the trust that we can facilitate a lot of our own healing on our own. How is it that animals know how to source plants to eat when they have certain ailments? Anyone with a dog has seen their sweet pet eat something in the field one day that they've never seen them eat before. Trust me, this isn't random hunger. Many, many animal species do this all the time, and precisely know the medicinal plants that their bodies require. They are in harmony with the quantum field that weaves their body with their mind and with their environment. To me, this is our natural state, and yes, this is a state that we've lost access to for the most part… but it's still there below the veil of the subconscious. Practices like Qigong, Meditation, Yoga, and the healing arts, when practiced consistently and with Heart-resonant intent, will enhance our natural Qi Effect and awaken the intelligence latent in the coherent waveforms that dance within the molecules of every cell in our body.

Within each cell of our body, wave functions describe the quantum field dynamics of covalent molecular bonds. Schrödinger knew this and was able to see that each wave function carries information about life-force itself. He referred to this information about life-force as "genetic" information, and understood that this was the natural way for the molecules within genes to communicate the code required to build proteins in each and every cell. This is what genes are doing 90% of the time: they program the production of proteins to be used throughout the body for nearly every function from metabolism to repair. Schrödinger stimulated the greatest minds of his time such as the Danish Nobel Laureate Neils Bohr and the German-American biophysicist Max Delbrük who deeply explored the emerging research in genetics within the context of quantum theory. Schrödinger also influenced Pascual Jordan, the German theoretical physicist who helped pioneer the principle of "matrix mechanics" to describe how energy jumps states. The concept of Bohr's "complementarity" proved that you couldn't measure the specific feature of something like an electron's mass and also know it's momentum. He proved this mathematically and showed that you also had to take into account the influence of the observer and the measurement device itself. In other words, his research showed that nothing exists on its own; everything is inextricably interwoven together in the quantum field. This actually drove Albert Einstein and others crazy as they had previously held that everything had precise, measurable qualities. Bohr said things could actually have two complementary measurements depending on the observer. Each of these luminaries began to understand how quantum field principles, no matter how disruptive they were, had to relate to life sciences and our very human bodies. This shows us that our mind is the "observer" and our body is the measurement device. Our health is the outcome of the experiment. Each of us is a complete laboratory of sorts, with everything necessary to affect the wave function describing our current state of being. When we remember this and our latent healing abilities, and then learn how to fully activate the Qi Effect, I believe we will regain what it means to truly be human and move into the next stage of our evolution. The only technology required is our Heart-resonant Intuitive Mind…

…yet I continue to have faith in science as amazing researchers are embracing the courage required to push these concepts within the confines of the scientific community. In 2019, research published in the World Journal of Stem Cells by Facchin, Canaider, Tassinari, Ventura, et al, showed how cellular microtubules act as oscillators capable of synchronization and swarming to generate mechanical and electromagnetic patterns that impact biomolecular recognition. In other words, there is a highly dynamic and intelligent interaction taking place within and between cells in our body that operates not at a biochemical level, but at an energetic level. This vibratory energy holds the secret of how our body heals, rejuvenates, and carries the actual intelligence about its ideal, healed state of being.

Another, even newer research paper from 2022 that Frederica Facchin is also author on, Cell Responsiveness to Physical Energies: Paving the Way to Decipher a Morphogenetic Code, states the following: "Compelling evidence is presented, showing that biological patterns are strongly embedded in the vibrational nature of the physical energies that permeate the entire universe. We describe biological dynamics as informational processes at which physics and chemistry converge, with nanomechanical motions, and electromagnetic waves, including light, forming an ensemble of vibrations, acting as a sort of control software for molecular patterning." This points to the exciting trend moving us to understand the energetic nature of the world around us and opening the door to new ways to look at healing, which should empower anyone interested in Qi.

Even if this all starts to feel intellectually challenging, trust me that I'm doing my best to not get too technical, but a little insight into science is necessary to fully grasp the essence of the Qi Effect.

Let's take a look at two more aspects of Quantum Physics that are key to uncovering the nature of the Qi Effect: the concept of "Complementarity" and the role of the observer. "Complementarity" is a core quantum physics principle, and means that we can't simultaneously know every single detail about something we are observing. A good example of complementarity is found in the Heisenberg's Uncertainty Principle: we can know the mass of an object but we can't simultaneously know its momentum. Complementarity means that there are typically pairs of data about an object, mainly relating to subatomic elements, that are not knowable at the same time. Of course this throws traditional physicists into a tailspin. They have a mindset that is based on being able to know everything about everything at the same time. Quantum physics says that this is impossible. It also says that the observer (i.e. the person doing an experiment) influences the outcome of the experiment. This really drives Newtonians over the edge. They have to believe that the world is material and immutable and that it will consistently follow the fundamental rules of physics whether someone is watching it or not. Quantum physics absolutely proves that to be false. The observer in any experiment is key to defining the outcome. We live in a reality where our perception - and the influence energetically of our thoughts and attitudes - deeply influences everything around us.

The critical factor of the observer becomes fundamental not only to Quantum biology, but to our lives as well. It's what I've been teaching in workshops for three decades now, and points to the Taoist genius when presenting "Yi" along with breath and movement to define Qigong practice. Yi is our intentional component, and celebrates the observer whether it is you doing your practice or you facilitating healing in someone else. This is our gift in being human: to understand the massive power intention has to affect the quantum field around us. This is in part why Quantum biology will bring a renaissance to healthcare in the future: it will return the individual back into the relationship in the healing process between doctor and patient.

There is one more core principle of Quantum Physics that is paramount to understanding the Qi Effect, known as "quantum tunneling." In 1963, a Swedish physicist named Per-Olov Löwdin presented a series of papers describing how subatomic elements can "tunnel" energetically from one region to another between what would otherwise, in traditional physics, be impossible. He actually describes this as a mechanism for DNA mutations and first coined the term "quantum biology."

The best way I've found to begin understanding quantum tunneling is to start by seeing things like protons and electrons as quantum energy fields. These quantum energy fields are coherent, and in their energetic vibration they carry information. Waves and fields of energy potential will act as a barrier for material objects whereas other waves of energy can pass through them. When waves of energy pass through other waves of energy, they effect the overall wave function of the field matrix itself. Up until the discovery of this quantum tunneling, everyone believed in the Newtonian concept of limits and barriers. Quantum tunneling proves that these boundaries are illusory, and that subatomic particles have always been passing through these barriers, which explains things like photosynthesis, which up until recently has eluded a complete scientific explanation. What we think of as "limits" have all been illusory explanations when in fact subatomic energy transfer and communication lies at the core of most all function in the biological world.

It is fascinating to even consider, as Löwdin proved, that a single subatomic element called a proton can display quantum tunneling by moving past an otherwise impenetrable barrier in, lets say, a molecular bond. This is not just abstract theory. Löwdin showed that tunneling past a molecule's hydrogen bond that joins DNA base pairs can create a mutation in that DNA's replication process that causes cancer. This is an absolutely new "energy-based" way to look at illness that offers fabulous healing potential. Science has come to accept that quantum tunneling is key to other scientific observations as well, such as nuclear fusion, nanotechnology, superconductivity, and even molecular cloud formation in the regions where stars are formed throughout the Universe. We are starting to understand that we have to move beyond traditional physics and biochemistry to explain our body and our world, and accept that we are a complex energetic wave function that is affected by the most subtle shifts in quantum vibration. The most influential of these shifts is our mind itself.

Quantum Biology is the real promise of understanding how our body/mind/spirit truly functions as an entangled whole, and will help Western medical science to finally accept that it is only by looking at our biological systems as a dynamic wave function that we can support true and lasting healing. More and more universities around the world, from Princeton in the U.S. to the University of Surrey in the U.K., are offering courses on Quantum Biology, so it is promising that cutting edge research will eventually break the stranglehold Big Pharma currently has on healthcare. I probably wouldn't have dropped out of medical school in the '70s if there was a Quantum Biology curriculum being taught. Instead, my Qigong and energy healing training back then took me on a more ancient route with Master elders from the East.

Dr. Peitre Gariaev, the amazing Russian researcher, took Quantum Biology to new levels in the early 1990s with his theories and repeatable experiments. They showed how the DNA in our cells acts like a coherent wave form. DNA actually carries and can transmit all the information required to heal other cells. In his groundbreaking experiments on laboratory rats with pancreatic cancer, he used a specially tuned laser to "harmonize" the frequency of a rat with a healthy pancreas. He and his team then directed this tuned laser beam to the rat with the pancreatic cancer. After a few treatments, the cancer went into remission, and with further treatments the rat's pancreas returned to a healthy state. Dr. Gariaev showed through repeated experiments such as this, that an "energetic signature" is transmitted at the DNA level of every cell. He went as far as to say that this was a "language" and that this information could be captured (stored) using the laser and then communicated (transmitted) with the same laser.

A research team in Canada heard about the work of Dr. Gariaev, who was nominated as a candidate to be considered for the Nobel Prize in Medicine in 2019, and invited him to come from Russia to replicate this experiment. He took up the offer and brought his laser set up to Canada where the highly scrutinized process was carried out with a team of medical researchers. To the Canadian's surprise, the experiment was successfully replicated and another rat was cured of pancreatic cancer.

You may find this to be very "edgy" science, but there is even more of Gariaev's cutting-edge work to discover in the next chapter. Sadly, there was also some suspicious activity at the Canadian lab when the research team left after the successful demonstration. It turned out that all of the specialized laser equipment was stolen along with Dr. Gariaev's scientific documentation. This is how threatening and disruptive breakthrough technology is to the established medical industrial complex.

We will dive deeper into how Gariaev's breakthroughs are so significant to both the world around us as well as our own self-healing potential. Know for now that his work shows how life-force, Qi, is not only infused into every cell of our body at the molecular level, but that the Qi Activation intelligence can be shared across the quantum field of the body through intention and focus. This is the essence of the Qi Effect.

What is really exciting is that these explorations continue to this day, and as I write, Carlo Ventura, MD, PhD and Professor of Molecular Biology University of Bologna, is doing amazing work to apply these concepts in practical ways. He is extremely credible as a trained Cardiologist and as Director of the National Laboratory of Molecular Biology and Stem Cell Engineering of the National Institute of Biostructures and Biosystems (NIBB) at the Innovation Accelerators of CNR, Bologna, Italy. His studies focus on stem cell vibration for healing and rejuvenation, and are similar to what Gariaev pioneered in Russia. Dr. Ventura is looking at DNA and cell reprogramming via epigenetic information delivered by magnetic fields, sound vibrations and coherent water. His studies aim at exploring cell biology in the light of physics, using magnetic fields, nanomechanical vibration, and light to develop a regenerative medicine protocol relying upon the features of these physical energies to allow reprogramming of tissue-resident stem cells. This strategy is paving the way for an approach to regenerative medicine executed without the need for cell or tissue transplantation, and based upon the enhancement of our innate, self-healing potential. As science begins to focus more on our body as an energetic matrix, healing solutions will begin to focus on using electromagnetic energy instead of surgery or pharmaceuticals. This is the inevitable merging of science with the Qi Effect principles and proves positively how we can activate Qi life-force energy using our natural abilities of mental intention, breathing, and specific body movement.

I have to mention the amazing work of Michael Levin, PhD, Distinguished Professor of Biomedical Engineering at Tufts University, is doing toward changing the way science looks at biology and combines developmental biophysics, computer science, and behavioral science to understand how cognition "scales up" from the metabolic and physiological competencies of single cells, to the organ-building and repair capabilities of cellular groupings and the whole organism itself. Basically, this "cognition" is the collective intelligence of the cells themselves that helps them navigate, function, reproduce in their morphogenetic and behavioral environments. His work is on the cutting edge of understanding the latent intelligence at the cellular level and how to tap into this to assist in areas as diverse as the regeneration of organs and limbs to repairing birth defects and cancer reprogramming. If this doesn't pique your interest into the importance of the Qi Effect, I'm not sure what will.

Activating life-force energy - Qi - is what empowers cells to actualize their "intelligence" and use the information programmed both genetically and energetically within their structural matrix. What Levin refers to as morphogenesis is what he calls "the ability of multicellular bodies to build, repair, and improvise novel solutions to anatomical goals." These "goals" are the basics of what keeps our bodies alive in the face of aging, stress, disease, and so forth. What Levin is doing - not unlike Gariaev - is showing that there is an intelligence at levels within our body that not only can be tapped, but activated and even guided. This is parallel to the principles of using our "Yi" in Qigong, using our mental focus and visualization to activate Qi. Levin is deconstructing the processes at the cellular and quantum levels that are in fact at work to make the structural and energetic shifts that will allow us to rejuvenate and heal our bodies in a future where we will live longer and healthier lives. If this is in fact possible as he is showing every day in the Levin Lab at Tufts where he has actually regenerated frog limbs, then we have proof of what the body is capable of if we can tap into this subconscious intelligence by activating Qi through practices such as Qigong.

Although this may all appear far-fetched, the basic process of photosynthesis that I mentioned before is a prime example Quantum Biologists use to demonstrate an obvious instance of how we need to change the way we look at biology and biochemistry. Photosynthesis allows plants and some bacteria to convert photons - in the form of sunlight - into life-force energy, and science has always attempted to explain photosynthesis in biochemical terms. However, Quantum mechanics is what finally has allowed us to understand the incredible wisdom taking place in every leaf of every plant you look at. In many ways, photosynthesis defies the standard biochemistry of plant biology because how a plant derives energy for a photon can't be fully explained without the idea that electrons can pass through otherwise resistant energetic barriers in the plant cell. The effects of quantum tunneling can oftentimes overcome very wide energy gaps between different states existing in molecular structures. Overcoming these energy barrier gaps that exist in biochemical environment don't make sense in standard scientific explanations, yet they enable living organisms to capture and store the energy carried from the Sun by photons. This leaves lots of room for exploring where Qi can fit in as a quantum biology explanation... and solution.

Let's return back to our own body. According to Löwdin, a proton can energetically "tunnel" and signal a shift in the coherent information field of DNA to affect critical cellular function. This is amazing, and cannot be explained solely through biochemistry or traditional Newtonian physics, which is why quantum biology will in fact be the future solution for understanding what actually gets us sick and creates illness… and what also keeps our bodies healthy and vibrant.

The insights we have gained from our dive into Quantum physics so far are:

1) Everything in and around us is made up of quanta (packets) of energy

2) This energy is held together through a field coherence that carries intelligence and information

3) Energy quanta regularly moves between this dimension and some other one

4) The observer plays a key role in all experiential outcomes

5) Waveforms, as energy quanta, "tunnel" through all apparent barriers

As we return to the Qi Effect, it seems quite consistent with what we know through Quantum physics and the ongoing research that continues to be done. We can see that our bodies, from their fundamental atomic structure to the electromagnetic energy field dancing around us, are a complex and intelligent coherent quantum field effect. Yes, you can describe your body in material terms or even biochemical terms, but we have come to learn that this is a very limited perspective that can't help us answer most of life's pressing issues. This limited perspective also reduces your possibility for healing and personal transformation.

Allopathic medical science is absolutely inept when it comes to chronic health issues. This ineptitude has led to pharmaceutical drug treatments that typically either sustain life in a slow decay of organ system breakdown, or simply expedite death. I know this sounds harsh, but please do your research as I have. Iatrogenic causes of death refers to deaths directly related to medication 'side' effects, hospital-acquired infections, treatment errors, surgical complications. Iatrogenic causes of death are extremely high. Johns Hopkins University did a study in May of 2016 stating that nearly 250,000 people die each year from iatrogenic causes. This study may not be exactly perfect and accurate, but we have to believe it is close to accurate. What's curious about this is that when you read about death rates in the 18th Century, it was only those who could afford medical treatment from doctors that were on the death rolls. Farmers, pioneers, ranchers, and people who lived naturally off the land were not the ones dying of disease.

Facts are facts, and I don't want to go much farther into this. But I do want to say that there are amazing physicians and nurses in the world, people who really care about the health and wellbeing of their patients. These are people who entered medicine for all the right reasons, took the ancient Hippocratic Oath, and from my experience, offer patients the least invasive solutions first. They also focus on early treatment protocols and healthy lifestyle, which include conscious eating, exercise, positive attitudes, stress management, empowering relationships, etc. All of this is critical to "thriving." Without these basics, all of the work you do to activate the Qi Effect will be for naught. I watch too many people coming to Qigong when they reach a critical stress point in their body, mind, and spirit health. They then put massive expectations on the practice of Qigong to "fix" them. I'm happy to see so many people who make amazing shifts in their lives and health even at this "last chance" attempt to regain their health, but think how much easier it would all be if we didn't wait until things got so bad?

Looking at the five Quantum Physics insights above, think about how the Qi Effect principles can be embraced and applied in your life. Remember that the first step in any change is to embrace a transformation in our belief system. Einstein, like so many of his contemporary wizards, was also a philosopher to one degree or another. He was supposedly attributed to saying, "We can't solve a problem with the thinking that created the problem." When we look at our five Quantum physics insights, see which ones challenge what you believe about yourself and life around you. Next, see if you can accept each concept in a way that you can practically apply it to your life. Just as the famous quantum theorists made the leap from hard science to philosophical explorations about life and humanity, you are being asked to embrace the very principles that are fundamental to life itself and weave them into how you see yourself in the mirror. Can you close your eyes and make the choice to see yourself in a new way? Can you see your Conduit nature and then embrace how you can tap into the infinite Qi field available to you? Can you accept that as an energy body, you have access to resources that you may not have realized or accepted before? Can you sense that the emerging science of quantum biology will help shift the way we all look at health and vitality… and that right now, you have the choice to begin that transformation within you?

The Qi Effect is the essential quantum explanation for how all matter comes into being in our dimension and how life emerging from that matter is sustained. Through what is known as dynamic quantum tunneling, the coherent waveforms we call subatomic particles are electromagnetic fields from this dimension that "tunnel" into the Qi Field and tunnel back again into this dimension quantumly entangled with Qi. All life as we know it is energized, sustained, and maintained through this amazing process.

There is a lot of research on the process of dynamic quantum tunneling, such as the paper by Stephan-Arlinghaus titled, "Dynamic Tunneling: Theory and Experiment" printed in March 2011. The paper shows that there is a quantum transport between regions that are classically not connected. Michael Wilkinson, in his September 1986 paper titled "Tunneling Between Tori in Phase Space," explains how this dynamic quantum tunneling can address the problem faced in subatomic movement between dimensions. As theoretical as all this may sound, every bit of this is applied to the cutting edge of atomic energy research.

Although there is much hope in cold fusion reactors to create safe electric power, it still seems a long way off and there are no practical applications at this point. Most atomic fusion is "thermonuclear" fusion, which means that the fusion of atomic nuclei generate energy and can only take place in an extremely hot environment. Tokamak facilities around the world have actually been attempting to do this for years, but it always takes more input energy than what is generated. Of course our Sun and most all stars in the Universe attain fusion naturally at a temperature of nearly 15 million degrees Fahrenheit because of their massive gravitational force pressing down on their hydrogen fuel. What we've discovered, though, is that this heat is not really enough to trigger the fusion reaction alone. It requires quantum tunneling to explain how it actually occurs. This takes us back to the last chapter when we explored how matter comes into this dimension in the first place, and we can see now that there is clearly energetic exchange, entanglement, and dynamic quantum tunneling occurring, most likely between the Qi Field life-force source and everything in our dimension.

In the realm of our daily "macro-level" life, we have more than enough to manage in our basic three-dimensional world. Fortunately this is a relatively stable domain and not much disappears or reappears that often, save our car keys or sunglasses when we are in a rush to find them. On the quantum level, the subatomic elements of the metal and plastic in your car keys and sunglasses are popping in and out of this dimension on a regular basis. No, this doesn't necessarily explain why you keep losing your stuff, but it does point to how the concept of "dimensional tunneling" takes on a different meaning at the quantum level.

Have you heard of the Tokamak? No, it's not from a science fiction novel, but it feels like it could be. Do some research and you'll discover that this acronym from the Russian language, where the first developments were made back in the 1950s by Soviet physicists Igor Tamm and Andrei Sakharov, describes a class of thermonuclear fusion reactors. Yes, there are working devices here on Earth that create a sustained atomic fusion reaction that is contained by a very powerful magnetic field, much like a star. This fusion reaction creates high-energy plasma that is held together in a torus shape by enormous magnets mirroring that shape. The torus is the donut-shaped geometry seen in the Earth's electromagnetic field that we discussed in the previous chapter. It is probably the most commonly seen geometrical shape in our Universe and expresses the balanced dynamics of electromagnetic flow. This is why the Tokamak reactor utilizes this torus shape, and even though it still takes more energy input that we get out of this reactor, research continues to this day. The common wisdom is that maintaining the torus shape of the energy field is key to success. Science knows the torus shape is reflected in everything from the energy field around every tiny atom to the giant accretion clouds emitted as light/space/time bending radiant energy surrounding every Black Hole. The torus is also seen in nearly everything in between, from the Earth's Van Allen Belts to the shape of apples and hurricanes. There is an energetic fingerprint of sorts in our Universe, and the torus just may be what that is. This continues to point to the fact that everything in our known world carries an energetic, electromagnetic field around it, mirrored fractally from the smallest to the largest resolution of granularity. Even many Qigong moves follow the shape of the torus, yet most instructors don't recognize this and were never taught it by their teachers. That the torus structure has at its core (the hole in the donut) a place of aligned, neutral harmony (just like the calm in the eye of a turbulent hurricane) is tribute to why these Qigong moves bring such inner peace and can so effectively active the Qi Effect. It is natural that we are driven by intuitive, subconscious Universal principles and we express these principles many times unknowingly. In the "Qi Effect Exercises" chapter of this book, you'll learn some of these types of Qigong moves and Spiral Breathing techniques that activate Qi by engaging the torus energetics, and experience for yourself how you feel from these empowering practices.

So you see, my task is to weave together real science and research that you may not be aware of and show that there could be a very simple way to explain this experience we call reality by accepting, on the deepest level, that everything is in fact energy, which is the essence of E=mc2: but energy with a much wider degree of freedom than we were taught. Accepting that, and then understanding how our thoughts so deeply influence this subtle world - and how the practice of interoceptive "inner awareness" - gives us a real pathway to personal empowerment, healing, freedom, and transformation.

Through quantum entanglement and field coherence, the amalgam of our atomic structure is known to be an integrated quantum field effect wave function, and works together as an intelligent whole. This information-carrying intelligence, held in part by coherent fields we know as molecules and specifically DNA, merges on the physical at the inception point of embryonic development, continuing through meiosis and mitosis in every cell. During the initial stages of womb gestation, our original embryonic cells were all stem cells. These pluripotent cells were not yet differentiated into specific types of cells such as liver, heart, bone, etc. They each carried the intelligence and data about the complete, whole, and perfect human body. In this pluripotency, the ability to become any and every type of cell, there is also a massive intelligence for not only carrying the complete genetic map of building a working human, but also carrying the Qi life-force consciousness necessary to sustain the building process itself. Consciousness itself is a field function following these same principles, and as such is entangled throughout every atom in the Universe. Each of us is an expression of this consciousness and life force, expressing the infinite magnitude of life-force through our personal, human experience. Learning to use the full capacity of our consciousness, we have the ability to activate the Qi Effect at higher rates of efficiency, moving us from a life of surviving to a life of thriving. Thriving is the ultimate expression of the design of our physical and energy body. When molecules, including those that make up our genes, are not suppressed by toxins or toxic situations, they can express their innate intelligence and vibratory resonance that leads to optimal health. This thriving is further optimized when we embrace a healthy lifestyle and a positive world view. The ultimate step in thriving is understanding the Qi Effect and learning to fully activate Qi.

Optimizing our body form and function activates the Qi Effect. Hurting and weakening our body form and function deactivates Qi Effect. This is why the ancient Taoists placed great emphasis on keeping our body healthy as they intuitively and experientially knew that activating the Qi Effect depends on the body's ability to be a conduit for Qi to be expressed. Taking care of our body temple through a healthy lifestyle optimizes our ability to activate the Qi Effect as our conduit nature at the molecular level opens the pathways to Qi activation.

Obviously if you pull a plant out by the roots or deprive it of sunshine and water you've deactivated the Qi Effect and it will soon die. You've cut off its ability to activate Qi. The same is true for our own body.

This also relates to our thoughts and emotions as they are energetic fields that create either enhancers or stressors for the body and Wei Qi field. Every thought we have, every emotion we express contributes to either activating the Qi Effect or deactivating the Qi Effect. The good thing about this is that we have a choice about the thoughts and emotions that we carry and express. The bad thing is that we forget we actually have this choice.

Emotion Alchemy is a technique that I've developed and teach around the world that transforms a Qi deactivating thought or emotion into a Qi activating one. It a strategic and conscious process that helps us slow down our observation and reactions so that identify how we sabotage ourselves without even realizing it, and in so doing, deactivate the Qi Effect. This ends up being expressed in some bodily symptom through any "weak link" in our immune system or physiology.

In Emotion Alchemy, we first analyze if an action needs to be taken on a thought or emotion. Is it an immediate issue that requires a response?

Can you do anything about it in this moment? If so of course, act on it. If not, then begin the transformation. Identify it as a Qi deactivating energy. Say thank you, from your Intuitive Mind, for observing this. Identify where originates; either the Survival Mind or Intellectual Mind. Next, return to the Intuitive Mind. There, your Heart resonance will see the difference between activating and deactivating and consciously choose activation of Qi. There's a fair bit more to this technique that involves the Traditional Chinese Medicine (TCM) Five Elements and Five Emotions and transforming survival-based emotions into empowered, Heart-centered emotions but I trust this gives you the idea of how activating the Qi Effect is truly a body, mind, and emotion process that we actually have a lot of influence over.

The ancient Chinese Taoists may have been a bit more "Container" oriented in their concepts of cultivating, gathering, and storing Qi than I am, but still we share the overarching concept that tapping into the Qi Effect through our personal energy field, called the Wei Qi field, is a positive and important thing to pursue. To the ancients, this energy field we now know as the toroidal electromagnetic field around both our bodies and every atom, is a "protective" field. Though they didn't use the term "immune system" in ancient times, they intuitively knew that developing the Wei Qi field would help keep a person healthy and build longevity. We now know through scientific research and research-supported data that our immune system is dramatically improved when our stress is reduced, and the effects of aging are diminished when chromatin telomeres in our cells are lengthened. Both stress reduction and telomere lengthening are shown in countless research studies to be exactly what occurs in the deep, abdominal breathing and slow movements of Qigong practice. Research, such as the 2021 study at the University of Glasgow by Nickolas MacKenzie that I participated in, shows that people can achieve and sustain the "Qigong State" (flow state) through regular meditative movement practice. Findings showed that somatic awareness, which typically involves conscious breathing, intentional slow movement, and positive mental focus, was consistently the first step in achieving this state. All related research concurs that a "Conduit" flow approach to well-being provides many beneficial results on a body, mind, and spirit level.

Qi is always "there" - anywhere and everywhere. Damaged or stressed body parts, tight muscles, inflammation, negative thinking, and more all disturb Qi activation efficiency. Optimized Qi activation is a combination of attending to physical/psychological alignment while using your intention, breath, and focus to "see" and influence the activation of Qi in your body and in the world around you.

Science is slowly moving away from reductionism and into holism and this is key to our evolution. Where reductionism looks at systems based on their component parts granularity for explanations and solutions, holism looks at how the systems actually influence the component parts. This may sound obvious, but it's easy to see how everything from allopathic medicine to corporate management operates from a very limiting reductionistic mindset. Component quality - like cell wellness in the body - is determined by the broader system. For living creatures, this "broader system" is the holistic, interwoven dynamic of the whole body, which includes our psychological, emotional, and electromagnetic energetic body. This is key to seeing how the Qi Effect is influenced - and it is best to see it holistically and not from a reductionistic point of view.

The Qi Effect is really a description of how our miraculous bodies and consciousness works. It truly holistically describes how all living creatures, from microscopic organisms to insects, plants, and mammals stay alive through the dynamic interrelationship between matter, electro-magnetic energy, and Qi. Since the basic function of life is to survive, most living creatures go from birth to death along a path of functional survival. Even apex predators in nature follow this trajectory of sustaining their species at a survival level. As humans, we have a curious feature of our consciousness that understands the difference between "surviving" and "thriving." We know this intuitively, and in the next chapter we will explore more about this and what it truly means to be an expression of Infinite Consciousness knowing itself through our own unique human experience. As for the Qi Effect, research and experience shows that this is our practical and tangible pathway to shift from just surviving and into truly thriving. Learning to become a conscious participant in fully activating Qi is the secret.

Our Three Minds

I imagine that after reading the title of this chapter, you're thinking about how having to deal with just one Mind on a daily basis is already a heavy load, so please don't burden me with two more… You may also be thinking that I'm about to reveal your latent schizophrenic nature. If you thought that, you're actually on the right path. You may have also jumped to the conclusion that one of these "Minds" is your subconscious Mind, while the third Mind is that one piece of the puzzle that you missed when you were last reading about Freud or Jung. We're actually not going in that direction, and I promise that we will tie these three Minds back into the Qi Effect.

The nature of being and of our existence is known as "ontology," and has been the fodder of philosophers since the beginning of time. Ontology has created many stable and long-lasting jobs for these philosophers, good careers where they can't ever really get fired for not doing their job because no one knows exactly what "the job" is. It's hard to fire them because it isn't possible to do a qualitative fact check on the work of a philosopher. While mathematicians and biologists are tested for real and measurable facts that define the level of their expertise, philosophers simply defer to other philosophers. It's like a big club where every philosopher watches the other's back. They make sure that they've all read the same books written by other philosophers and can quickly quote anything any other philosopher said or wrote. Whether or not they really agree is beside the point.

When someone can't prove you right or wrong, you have very high job security. As a result, philosophers have maintained their long lineage since the days of Nineveh originating in 6,000 B.C. Unlike the good, salt-of-the-earth blacksmiths and candle makers that have fallen to the wayside in recent centuries, philosophers continue to maintain the very job security they had in those days of Ashurbanipal's library and lecture circuit in and around the Fertile Crescent of Mesopotamia.

I've taken you on the philosopher's journey because in order to explore the nature of "Mind," we must explore the essence of ontology. To know the nature of our being and very existence, we must know the origin of consciousness. Who are "we" but that which knows ourself to be. This "self knowing" is called sentience and it is what most philosophers require in order to have anyone around actually willing to listen to them. To be sentient is what separates us from animals and rocks, horseshoes and candles. At least that's what we're told. I'll get into that issue shortly, but for now let's say that only humans are sentient, and as such, they have the "self knowledge" to be aware that they are humans. This awareness comes from consciousness, and consciousness precludes the basic working of something that we call "the Mind."

We have been told that our "Mind" is precious: do you remember those 1970's TV ads where they showed eggs frying in a hot skillet that pushed the slogan, "A mind is a terrible thing to waste"? We all heard "Make up your mind!" incessantly when we were teens, didn't we? Then there was "Mind your manners." John Lennon sung us his great hit, "Mind Games." These days, we're inundated with the push to be "mindful." I could go on but you get the idea.

The big question remains, "what is this Mind anyway?" Most people will say, "Well silly, it's… you know, the part in your brain you think with." Then most everyone in the room, except maybe the philosophers, will nod knowingly before someone conveniently changes the subject to save any further torture and asks who wants to go with them to Starbucks.

We are in a world where we simply assume what Mind is. Sadly, most of us have lost the ability to do anything other than ignore and change the subject. At best, we manage the Mind in the way we would manage a pet or a garden. We do everything we can with this Mind to keep it on track, to keep it busy, to make sure we take it out for walks or weed it regularly. We show off when it can do a trick and we get upset when it pees on the carpet. Whoops, did I mix up "mind" and "pet"? Sorry about that, maybe I switched them around because that's how I see most people are dealing with their own Mind.

For those of us who practice meditation, we've grown familiar with the phrase "Monkey Mind." I watch people use it as an easy excuse for their "busy, unfocused, and unmanageable" thoughts that jump from branch to branch like a monkey. Monkeys are actually very focused at survival skills. As humans, our intellect is focused to the point of becoming rigid, and the excuse of a "monkey mind" moment misses the point of what we are actually experiencing in our Mind. While living in Beijing, I loved attending the Chinese classical theatre performances. My favorite performances featured the Monkey King. Like the theater of Ancient Greece, these performances are designed to help the audience understand human nature in the guise of entertainment. Every time, the clever Monkey King gets himself into trouble just like our Mind does when we don't understand it. None of the Emperor's best warriors could beat the Monkey King in combat or keep him from sneaking past the palace guards, symbolizing that the Mind can't be controlled by force. Each theatre performance ends the same way. After countless wins by the Monkey King, he finally becomes subdued by the Buddha's hand: a 10 meter long, upward facing golden palm prop that slides from off stage to center stage. This Buddha's hand represents the deep peace of Heart energy, the surrender of meaningless desire and the return to our Buddha nature. The Monkey King shakes and jumps around, pleading with the audience to help him. Finally, he sheepishly crawls onto the golden hand of the Buddha and curls up in a fetal position. The curtains close as the large Buddha hand begins its slow slide off-stage with the subdued Monkey King finally at peace.

The Chinese portrayal of the Monkey King shows us how gently guiding the unruly parts of our Mind back into Heart Resonance meets with far greater success than trying to attain control by way of force. Those of us who practice Qigong and the Taoist arts know that the center of the palm is where the powerful Heart resonant, "Lao Gong" acupuncture point is located. Translated as "ancient discipline," this point in our hand lies on the "heart protection" Jing Mai (energy meridian channel) leading directly to the Pericardium which covers and protects the physical heart in each of us. The ancient Taoists had such great insight...

Though the ancients in most cultures around the world felt that the Mind was centered in the heart, we in the modern world have been conditioned to believe that our Mind is situated in our brain. It's supported by most mainstream science since if there is neurological damage to the brain, our mental ability is thusly affected. Massive amounts of money have been invested over the years to map the human brain to understand exactly what cognitive function occurs where. During the Obama Administration, an enormous US$4.5B initiative was undertaken to map the brain. Since all of the money went to known players in the "material science club," nothing was discovered that wildly surprised anyone. The research was constricted by a purely mechanical perspective of the brain and its functions as any electronically wired computer would be deconstructed. One important discovery is that there are over 100 billion neurons in the brain and even more glial cells, all of which play critical roles in inter-neural communication even though we still don't understand their full function. It is wonderful that we learned more detail about the neural pathways and the physiological connections that define brain function, however that limited mechanical view of brain research is more akin to learning how an automobile is built than how to actually drive it.

Driving the brain is actually the domain of Mind.

Brain is not Mind.

Mind is not brain.

I want to make sure we get that clear. Sure, if you damage a specific part of the brain that is associated with "memory" then you will have issues accessing certain types of memories. Damage another part of the brain that deals with analytical function and the ability to calculate a math equation will be impaired. The question is, has the Mind been affected... or was it simply the pathway to access the Mind that was affected? Research and conjecture increasingly demonstrate how the brain is more like an antennae or a field generator than a storage facility. Some even claim that memories are not directly stored in our gray matter, but rather are "accessed" by our neural networks from the quantum field, or what the ancient Hindus referred to as the "Akasha" (where the term Akashic Records is derived from) which points to the universal field all around us.

We have also discovered over the past decades that the exact brain cells that are in your skull also appear in your abdominal region. That old adage "trust your gut" carries a lot of weight knowing this. Actually, neurons are distributed throughout the spinal cord and elsewhere in the body, so this whole idea of Mind/Body wisdom starts to take on a deeper and deeper sense of truth.

So "where" is Mind amidst all this random distribution of neurological concentration around the body? And how is it that people who suffer damage to specific parts of the brain can learn to "think around" the damaged areas and defy scientific logic that claims this shouldn't be possible?

Mainstream science, whether it's the biochemists or the physicists, have a difficult time letting go of the idea that everything is physical and tangible. It is this very rigid world view that ties the scientific community to believe that Mind has a physical, typically brain-centric origin. As long as this is the common view, and what college students get tested on to graduate, we will perpetuate a very limited and deceptively wrong view of Mind. As we discussed in the last chapter, the emergence of Quantum Biology is the field of science that will help us merge "matter" and "Mind" in a way that will help make sense of so many currently contradictory aspects of why we have disease and why it is so difficult to heal.

Some people jumped on the bandwagon a few years ago to call the gut the "second brain" and as such, the second Mind. Although that disrupted the clear delineation of brain-and-body, most people in the scientific community quietly reconciled this and went back to their microscopes. Then we had the research of Russian scientist Dr. Peitre Gariaev who's groundbreaking quantum biology work shows that our DNA not only carries a very stable and coherent electromagnetic quantum field, but it also leaves an energetic imprint on its environment, in the background field of seemingly empty space. DNA, which of course is only seen scientifically in its molecular (tangible) form with apparently clear biochemical functions, is actually a very stable energetic waveform according to Gariaev. It acts through specific design oscillations and coherent acoustic and electromagnetic fields that the atoms and molecules that make up the DNA create. This shows that there is not only "information" held in the quantum field of the DNA, but arguably, an active intelligence. The implications of this research (which I get into deeper in our chapter on Epigenetic Qi) is that yet another "Mind" exists in every cell in our body since there is DNA in the nucleus of every single cell.

Curiously, Dr. Gariaev passed away suddenly after he started speaking publicly about how his findings and low-cost health solutions would lead to the end of Big Pharma. This was in November of 2019, and just one month before SARS-COv2 emerged on the scene. To add to the curious nature of all this, after his death, his wife made public a letter he received from the Nobel Prize Committee informing him he was a candidate for the coming year's Nobel Prize for Science. Hmmm…

So yes, the Mind is a terrible thing to waste…

Yet as we can see, there is less and less scientifically provable evidence that "Mind" is trapped in the brain, or in neurons elsewhere in the body, or even in cells throughout the body. What we are led to grasp is the concept that "Mind" is not constrained to any physical or spacial location. If Mind can express through neural/glial networks in the brain and in neural concentrations in the gut and in the vibratory quantum field of DNA, then why can't Mind express itself in the Qi Field that permeates our body and extends beyond the body itself?

In one of the early chapters of this book, I did my best to discuss not only a simple but radically new view of cosmology, the creation of our Universe, but to also discuss the energetic structure of atoms. I know some of you wish I would just race past all this science and just talk about all the feel-good subjects like how we are all connected as one, how Love is the essence of all creation, and how we can heal ourselves on a body, mind, and spirit level. For you, please bear with this flow. Know that your patience radiates an intention out into the Universe and embraces an inclusive space for everyone...

...including those who really want to hear this science so that they can try and debunk me and call it quasi-science and then crawl back into their cave and rub their hands together feeling that they've secured another win for the "truth." I see these types the same way Galileo saw the Earth-centrists: the ones who either absolutely believed that the Earth was the center of the solar system, or they went along with it so that they could keep their jobs in government or in church-funded universities. Sadly, some things never change when fear influences and constricts our Mind.

...and yes, we will be getting to the Three Minds very soon... it just took all this to get there... but there is still one more thing...

There is one more group that would like to hear "the science," those beautiful souls whose intellects shine like a bright light. You know them, and maybe you are one of these, the ones who read the New York Times

Best Seller List each year and see how many of them they've read. I have two dear friends like this (believe it or not) and out of the last list of 100, they read around 95 of those books. I'm not sure I read that many books in my whole life, no less in one year! I think it's fabulous that people can read that much… and it's wonderful that it satisfies their need for knowledge and for being connected to the world around them.

With all this talk about "where" the Mind is, I will now share my view on "what" the Mind is. I won't just dive into the fact that we are Infinite Consciousness (Universal Mind) knowing itself through our Human Experience, not just yet at least. I think we need to first focus on the Mind that we can all relate to on a day-to-day basis.

The Mind we interact with every day is a very practical resource, and quite diverse. As we discussed in the beginning of this chapter, it's what provides us with sentience: self knowing. It's also what we use to decide what to purchase at the market, and who to be friends with. It's amazing how absolutely functional it is. It also gets really mixed up when certain tough choices need to be made, and it can make critical miscalculations that cost us lots of money and emotion from time to time. Yes, the same Mind can do all that and more.

What I feel is critical to achieve though, is a practical view of this otherwise amorphous thing we call Mind. This has helped me as a model to know myself better… and with the hundreds and hundreds of people I share this model with it provides a language for describing why we end up in some of the aforementioned messes that the Mind can get us into…

Instead of just describing Mind as Mind, I see it as three distinct bandwidths, much the same way the old radios were separated into frequencies to define each radio station. These bandwidths are:

Survival Mind

Intellectual Mind

Intuitive Mind

Without these clear distinctions, most people deal with life in very inefficient ways. It's much like using the wrong tool for a job and wondering why the task is such a hassle. Using a wrench for a job requiring a screwdriver can be frustrating, right? So what are these Minds anyway?

Survival Mind is a good place to start. It's that bandwidth, or portion, of our total Mind/consciousness that is allocated for all things having to do with our most basic survival needs and drives. In brain science we associate this with the "old brain" or the "reptilian brain" involving the amygdala and brain stem since these are primitive parts of the brain humans that have been carried with us from our earliest stages of evolution. Your Survival Mind isn't "housed" in these areas of your brain, but instead is "channelled" through these organic structures. Every thought you have about what you are going to have for lunch, how you are going to pay for your meal, and if what you ate was really good for you all originates in the Survival Mind. It's the frequency of your amazing Mind that hones in on everything that resonates with your home and community, and how you see yourself in relationship to others. It's the part of your Mind that reacts when there is a fire whether it is on your grill, in the forest, or in your passion.

When we are in Fear, we only see in limited ways. This Survival Mind reaction reduces the option set for solutions to such a small number that we feel trapped and typically sense danger and imminent failure/death. It's a wonderful observation when we can catch this in ourselves so that we can consciously shift out of this ancient conditioning and not fall prey to it...

The next Mind bandwidth is the Intellectual Mind. It is a bit more rarified than the instinctual Survival Mind as it relates to your intellect and analytic nature. This includes everything you know or think that is based on fact, detail, and judgement. We were taught that your "left brain" was where analytical thinking and calculations occurred. Think of this as at least part of your Intellectual Mind, or at least where your Intellectual Mind interfaces. This mental bandwidth is also where you process judgement, as this aspect of mind "weighs and balances," and therefore puts everything in your personal and social database into a hierarchical scale of likes and dislikes. The Intellectual Mind function is what is mostly fed in our academic education and is thus the most revered in the scientific world.

The third and final bandwidth, the Intuitive Mind, is the blessing we have that keeps us all from either killing each other or arguing all the time as the other two Minds battle for prominence within us. Well, that may be a bit dramatic, but the fact is, the Intuitive Mind doesn't obsess with survival nor does it engage in intellectual pursuits. You may ask what good is it then? That question shows how conditioned we are to put the Survival and Intellectual Minds so much in control of our lives. The Intuitive Mind is a bandwidth not easily mapped into the physical brain, although you may take a stretch and associate it with the Pineal region and insula area of the brain. If I was forced to create a body-map, I would rather associate the Intuitive Mind with the quantum field of the DNA matrix. This makes a lot more sense to me, and hopefully you will agree as we continue. The Intuitive Mind is that bandwidth that is widest of all, yet used the least for most people. It extends into the farthest access we have as humans to what the ancient Hindus called the Akasha, which simply can mean "outside" in Hindu. This is like the ancient Chinese Taoist word we spoke of earlier in this book, "wei" which also means "outside." The Intuitive Mind is the bandwidth of Mind we can use to access information that is both outside of our survival-based conditioning and outside of the database we carry intellectually. It can be best looked at as the ancients did, calling it Heart Mind (wisdom), as it is in alignment with Heart Resonance. Intuitive Mind defies space/time as it can provide us with amazing solutions that many times don't make logical sense in the moment, and that's why it is best associated with the Taoist Shen Qi, or "spirit energy."

In this way, the Intuitive Mind is much better at surviving than the Survival Mind… and much better at intellectualizing than the Intellectual Mind. I know, this appears very counter-intuitive, but you'll see how this ties into the Qi Effect and hopefully you will have that "aha moment" that the ancient Greeks referred to as a "metanoia." Metanoia simply means "a change in Mind." What I'd like to inspire in you is a "change in bandwidth" as the Mind itself is fine and there's really nothing we need to change… except which of our three bandwidths we allow to rule us.

If the Intuitive Mind is better at survival issues, why in the world would we relegate the Survival Mind to those duties? Well first, no one ever taught us that we even had a specialized Survival Mind, remember? We were only told that we had a "Mind." Back to the tool analogy, it would be like having a repair job to do in your kitchen and then dumping your whole tool box on the ground and staring at the pile of wrenches and screw drivers and hammers and pliers. Randomly, you grab at one tool or the other and start poking it at the leaky faucet wondering why the water was still dripping. If you didn't know what the right tool for the task was, you would waste a whole lot of time experimenting until you made a good fit and stopped the leak. By then, your kitchen floor would be flooded.

The second reason we use the Survival Mind for survival duties is because that's simply how we've been conditioned. If everyone obsesses with the struggle for survival the same way, then it must be right, right? In the West, we are typically taught the basic Puritanical principles of working hard to make a decent living. I have many Asian friends who don't have Puritanical European roots so they just use a different name for this type of conditioning from their parents and families that describes the same thing (usually it's Confucian.) These are epigenetically programmed in us and we will go into that important topic in the next chapter. What this means is that these survival drives are deeply embedded into every cell in our body. Our human bodies actually evolved and changed over 100,000 years based on this programming. Think of all our physical features that got selectively chosen based on our ability to better survive. This Mind-frequency bandwidth is deeply mapped into us. Of course we would rely on this automated response energetic to make most every decision about our survival. The curious thing is that in the 21st Century, we have very little in common with our primitive ancestors, yet we still rely on much of the same mental bandwidth to make decisions. Isn't it strange that the same Survival Mind that drove a cave dwelling mother to protect her offspring from Sabertooth Tigers by making a fire near the cave opening is the same Mind bandwidth a mother uses today to turn on the electric space heater when it gets cold in the family nursery?

The Intuitive Mind is also much more adept at the thinking we normally relegate to the intellect. How could this be, you say. Our Intellectual Mind bandwidth is perfectly honed and exercised in all thought processes that require analytical thinking, judgement calls, and precise measurement of the world around us. Well, it is fine-tuned for this type of thinking, but it still doesn't make it the best Mind bandwidth to use, at least not all the time. How many times did you find yourself in a jam, where you just couldn't get the answer to something that you'd been struggling over for hours? You've got a challenge at work, a task that needs to get done, but you simply can't come up with the solution. You go home thinking about this problem and with all your Intellectual Mind focused on this challenge, there seems no answer. You start getting frustrated. You start feeling anxious as your boss is depending on you. Your Survival Mind begins intruding on the process as begin to worry about your job and thereby your very livelihood. Stress continues to build and so you lie in bed unable to sleep. Exhausted, the good soldiers of your Intellectual and Survival Mind finally giving up and you begin to drift... Somewhere in this haze something comes to you, like a whisper. It's blurry at first, but something pops through into focus. What you see is the solution to your task at work. It seems so simple. It seems so obvious. It actually will work. You know it and write it down on a notepad, falling back asleep exhausted.

This is how the Intuitive Mind plays its role in our life. Typically it plays out like that little story. When all else fails and all your valiant attempts to "think through" a challenge fail, when you allow, once again, your Intellectual Mind and Survival Mind "bullies" to dominate your thinking, it is your Intuitive Mind that quietly rises up from the chaos and presents a solution.

We all know this process, we've all had these amazing insights in our life. Like the time you lost your house keys, and you were a wreck. You looked everywhere. You accessed (unknowingly) your Intellectual Mind to think through all the places you could have placed them. You thought and though and did your best to logic it out. Then your Survival Mind jumped into action and pushed you into overdrive, noting that if you don't hurry up and find those keys it would cost a lot of time and money to replace them... and if you can't drive your car then how are you going to work, and, and, and. Your Intellectual Mind and Survival Mind are simply doing the best they can do in this situation... and still you have no answer.

You allowed theses bullies to run the show while your Intuitive Mind has been sitting there in the wings, waiting. The Intuitive Mind is that bandwidth of your thinking process that is quite present in its functioning, extremely expansive in its scope, and in full access to most all memories and data that have come through your awareness at one point or another. Believe it or not, it also has access to information that did not actually come through your conscious awareness. This is because this bandwidth of Mind is not limited to the narrow frequency of information that we've been conditioned to know the world through. Yes, it can tap into the Qi Field, the quantum vibratory field, through which all information is entangled on a quantum level. These things are not accessible to your Intellectual or Survival Mind, and is the reason why you still can't find your keys.

So when you finally are so frustrated from beating your head against the problem of your lost keys, you stare out the window and wonder what your life will look like as it collapses under the weight and drama of this awful situation. You keep staring out the window while convincing yourself that you've done everything possible, and so you give up trying to figure it out. Life is over as you know it. And then your Mind drifts… You have some random thoughts, and you notice a bird sitting in the tree outside your window. The bird is a pretty blue color… yeah, the same blue color as that new ceramic vase you just purchased… oh my!!! The same vase that you inadvertently threw your keys into in the mad rush after you opened the front door with an armload of groceries just as the phone was ringing and your dog was barking as he knocked over your favorite potted plant and you were generally overwhelmed and not paying attention to details. It wasn't your Intellectual Mind paying attention, and your Survival Mind wasn't paying attention either. Both of them were completely consumed with attending to the chaotic hands full, phone-ringing, dog barking situation. And during all of this, your Intuitive Mind observed the entire scene clearly and wholly. The Intuitive Mind isn't preoccupied with the limitations that define the other Mind bandwidth bullies. Your Intuitive Mind saved the day once again… and you rush over to find your keys inside the vase, a place you'd never placed them before, leaving your "normal" bandwidth no point of reference to remember by.

What was that quote attributed to Albert Einstein? "You can't solve the problem with the thinking that created the problem." (It turns out that he actually never said this and later in this book I'll reveal who did :). The "thinking" that typically solves the unsolvable problems is done via the Intuitive Mind. It's also the bandwidth of your Mind that is your most amazing healing resource.

I trust that you are starting to get a feel for why it is so useful to have these Three Minds through which to understand all of your different thinking styles. Sure, it's a bit oversimplified but sometimes the best solutions are the ones where we can deconstruct complexity into tangible, bite-sized elements. As long as we keep believing that we have to "quiet our Mind" or continue saying that "our Mind keeps getting in the way" without knowing which bandwidth of Mind we are talking about, we will continue in the endless loop of not understanding our true nature. We'll keep losing our keys on a regular basis, and we will never be able to fully activate the Qi Effect.

It is a curious journey to begin languaging and observing the identification of the Survival, Intellectual, and Intuitive Mind. Some say that they feel a "forced" sense when asked to think about this, but that is only because their awareness and "thinking" is still lodged primarily in the Intellectual Mind. Our Intellectual Mind is not bad at all and plays an important role in our life, but being so distanced from Heart Resonance it is far from the operating frequency of the Intuitive Mind. As our Intuitive Mind is allowed to take more of a stand and becomes the awareness process for actually identifying Mind roles during self observation, the experience becomes softer and not at all forced. It becomes more like listening to music and noticing an oboe, and then a violin... a gentle awareness...

Remember too that only a fraction of Mind resides in the brain... and even saying this is a stretch. Mind consciousness is distributed throughout the atomic structure of the human body with higher probabilities of coherence in the DNA quantum field matrix itself within each cell's nucleus. Mind also resides outside your body, yes, your Mind is part of the field resonating around your physical structure, and extends throughout the Universe via quantum entanglement to varying degrees. This might seem pretty far-fetched, useless and impractical. You'd be amazed at how well this is corroborated with modern physics, let alone that this has been held to be true since ancient times. For those willing to explore this, and to stop being bullied by your Survival and Intellectual Mind, life will dramatically change for the better.

You may be wondering now about our subconscious Mind and where that plays into all this. Good question, and although we will get into this deeper in the next chapter on Epigenetic Qi, I'll touch on it here...Back in the '70s when I left my pre-med University training to study with an elder Master in Hawaii, I was very curious about the subconscious and its role in creating the chaos I saw in people all around me. Since early childhood I had watched how driven people were by motives that they weren't even aware of. I watched their anger, fear, grief, anxiety, worry… it all seemed so overwhelming for them. I could see that something invisible was driving them through situations and relationships that they seemed to have no control over. I regularly watched this in adults and was fascinated, especially when I tried to talk with them about and they told me that I didn't understand. I had been meditating since I was 7 or 8 years old, and remember getting insights into thoughts, beliefs, and emotions that sat in the shadows of people's Minds. I would watch as these energies influenced people without them even being aware of what was taking place. There were many times that I would help adults with challenges like grief at a funeral I attended, doing my best to explain that the sadness was beautiful to feel while the uncontrollable sobbing, anger, and anxiety was probably something that they could release once they really understood more about how none of us are just physical bodies. Who wants to hear a grade-school kid tell them something sensible… Fortunately, my family knew I was a bit strange, so they typically listened and even asked for advice (or maybe they were just spooked, who knows).

I remember the only time I ever saw my parents argue loudly in front of me and my six younger brothers and sisters at the time. At 8 years old I was shocked to see these two adults actually yelling at each other, they were my parents! Being the eldest and already handling tons of baby-caring duties, I felt we were a team that required peace, love and harmony. I remember watching for a minute or so as these two passionate, young Italians exchanged heated words. Then I yelled to get their attention… and I began to lay into to them that this was terrible behavior and they had no right to be like that to each other or to their kids. I remember all the babies just sat there and looked at me, then they looked at our parents, and then back to me again. My parents froze in that beautiful but awkward silence when you know you can't say anything to change the situation. I remember telling them, in no uncertain terms, to kiss, say you love each other, and promise that this would never happen again. They did, bless their Hearts. When the babies saw this, they all went about their business, playing and doing what they were doing. I never talked to my parents about this ever again, and they dare not bring it up to me either.

I wondered what force took over my parents in that moment. I was really too young to know about financial pressures that my Dad was under to feed 9 people every single day. I didn't fully understand the immense responsibility my Mom was under to take care of 7 kids, 4 who were in diapers at the same time. What I did know was that something came out of the shadows of my parents Minds that was very different than what I had seen before.

This was one way that I learned about the subconscious and came to understand that not only these overt outbursts like yelling and fighting came from this hidden region of Mind, but so did a major percentage of what we do and think every day. I learned this deeply from the elder Master I studied with for years in Hawaii. He had been a vibrant young doctor when he personally studied with Sigmund Freud in Austria, and later with Carl Jung. As a medically trained psychiatrist, this gave him deep insight into the exploration of the subconscious, as well as the collective unconscious. I was a sponge and absorbed all I could.

What this Master helped me understand, besides humbleness and how not to be so judgmental, was that there was an energetic nature of Mind and that it was truly linked into the quantum field. I lived in his clinic those years during my studies, which was Queen Liliuokalani's summer home on Oahu, Hawaii. My teacher had a suite upstairs, and I had my room off the lanai on the ground floor where I could welcome guests and patients that showed up at all times of day and night. There was a gardenia that seemed to be in constant bloom, and I felt like those unending blossoms were the gift the Universe blessed me with to deal with the general chaos of living in a working healing clinic.

During the many, many sessions that I would attend with this Master healer, I came to understand more and more about the subconscious

Mind and its energetic nature. I came to terms with the fact that humans are not simply biological robots driven by a chaotic array of biochemical interactions, and are in fact expressions of consciousness: individual points of attention of a vast and infinite Mind. This started to help me understand how each of us is so influenced by the energies around us, especially those that we are not even aware of that come from other people and even the Qi-infused quantum field around us.

This was big. This took Mind out of the neurological, biochemical realm and into a much more sensible perspective that could not only help me explain human behavior more efficiently, but it also provided real and lasting solutions to solve emotional, spiritual, and even physical challenges. The subconscious component, the part of our thinking and drive that we are not fully aware of, is what influences people more than they realize. Of course you can't "know what you don't know," which addresses the idea of being subliminally influenced every minute of our lives and not even realizing it. This goes for the conditioning we get bludgeoned by from the news media, to things we hear during the day that we don't register consciously. Subliminal Advertising was a phrase coined in 1957 and the concept was used in short films that they used to run before a movie started in public movie theatres. Single-frame images of a candy product or soda drink would be inserted in a film scene of two people talking and laughing and no one watching would consciously be aware that they saw that inserted image… but they had a sudden urge to get up and purchase candy and a soda. This is the manipulative power of this technique, and why the Supreme Court in the U.S. actually ruled against a company that said it was within their right of "free speech" to insert these messages. Although there are no laws against this in the United States (surprise?) the UK and other countries do in fact have laws against this subliminal messaging practice. I have to insert here another curious fact you may not be aware of: the pharmaceutical company advertising that is so prevalent in the United States and Canada is forbidden in most every other country in the world. Think of those TV commercials that you've seen showing a happy couple walking through a garden, smiling and holding hands, while the voice-over narrator is telling you the horrendous medical side effects and even death that will occur if you take the very drug they are advertising. If that isn't "subliminal" I'm not sure what is…

So, whether you live in countries where this type of mental manipulation takes place or not, trust me, you are constantly being delivered information and messages that enter your subconscious without your faintest notion. We have actually been conditioned to simply discount this, and I am amazed at how adept people are at holding a conversation when the TV or radio is blaring in the background. Modern overwhelm has taught people to filter out background chatter and all of this sadly and efficiently goes directly into the subconscious.

So where exactly is the subconscious you ask? Again, modern neuroscience has very clear ideas as to which various parts of the brain 'light up' under observation by using an fMRI scanning device in a lab. The fact is, as a recent Psychology Today article stated, "There are multiple neural correlates of consciousness, but we have not identified with certainty which ones are necessary and sufficient for consciousness." So, if the most well-funded researchers in the world can't even get the slightest handle on "consciousness" (remember how much the Obama Administration spent on all this), how in the world will they ever understand "sub-consciousness?" The very interesting thing here is that no one can say I'm wrong, mostly because they can't prove that they are right. The subconscious is up for grabs, but I trust you will find the next chapter very revealing as it relates to this in a very deep way…

For now, let's assume that there is a "subconscious" component to the Survival Mind and the Intellectual Mind. This makes sense, right? You know when you are driven to do something without thinking, like when a father jumps in front of a moving car to save his daughter. No time for conscious thought when survival is at stake, whether it is you or someone you love. On the flip side, there is the situation when everything seems to be going fine at the bar and then someone accidentally spills a drink on you and you immediately go into a rage and call them an idiot. A complete subconscious drive triggered the automated reaction that you were being attacked… and as soon as you see that it was an elderly blind woman who accidentally slipped when she spilled her drink on you, you realize how totally inappropriate your reaction was. What she is doing in the bar in the first place is for the Intellectual Mind to deal with…

For the Intellectual Mind, identifying its subconscious component is somewhat more complex as much of the Intellectual Mind operates under conscious direction. You know, when you are given a task to complete, an equation to solve, a book to read, things like that. Yet, even with the intellect, we have massively prepackaged conditioning that is called up from memory. This memory is not exactly "consciously" acquired, it just seems to appear… yes, like out of the subconscious. We also have incredible innate databases of scales and measurements, hierarchical and relational value systems, and acquired judgements. Some of these subconscious influencers have overtones of the Survival Mind, but they tend to get allocated to the Intellectual Mind when we espouse our knowledge to someone at a party we are trying to impress.

So we can see how Survival Mind and Intellectual Mind swap dominance in our thinking process quite naturally. They are like tag-team wrestlers, right? Those two characters who go into the fighting ring together and take turns, or work together, to beat the opponent. This happens at both the conscious and subconscious level.

We have the Survival Mind and the Intellectual Mind that we are somehow navigating through every moment of our life, and then there is also the subconscious component of both of them vying for a position depending on how they get triggered in different situations. Yes, it sounds a bit like a rodeo or a bad television situation comedy. Try to convince me that it is any different! You watch the world around you. You watch your own life. How can it be any different even if you have learned skills like coping mechanisms, accepted cultural behaviors, religious morals, or maybe even Qigong and meditation?

The answer is the Intuitive Mind.

The Intuitive Mind is the only bandwidth of consciousness/awareness that is in resonance with the Heart. Read that again and take it in because it's super important.

I can feel your Intellectual Mind immediately jumping on that statement like a hyena facing a pack of wildebeest. You have to try and convince yourself that you are mostly Heart-centered at work when you do the job you love. You also try to explain how your Survival Mind is full of Heart when you collect your paycheck. Please, don't humor me. This doesn't seem like Heart resonant flow...

To be Heart-centered is to be Heart resonant. This means that you are vibrating at the frequency of Heart space. Maybe a less flowery way to say that is that you are being directed by Heart energy. The ancient Taoists may say that your Wei Qi Field (energy field) is in resonance with your Heart vibration and as such, your Qi is being activated at that frequency. Taoists would also relegate this to Shen Qi, or the spirit aspect of self. So what is this Heart Resonance and why is it in this chapter about the Three Minds? I wondered when you were going ask...

First, notice that when I write "Heart" with a capital "H" I am talking about the energetic resonance, and when I type "heart" with the lower case "h" I am referring to the beating organ in your chest. The same goes for other words you see capitalized in the midst of a sentence, I am referring to their energetic/metaphoric nature rather than their existence as an object in the physical world.

To the wisdom holders of ancient times all around the world, Heart and Mind were synonymous. Even the term "Heart Mind" was common. In Classical Chinese Medicine, the brain wasn't even considered an organ in the way the stomach, liver, or heart was and the brain had no real role in thinking or the mind. The role of thinking was a function reserved for the

Heart. The concept of Shen Qi, that can be loosely understood as "spirit life force energy," was also associated with Heart Qi. This is where we drew upon consciousness and our mental functioning. Heart wisdom whas that sense of presence that tapped into a Universal sense of knowledge and essence. For the ancient Greeks, love associated with this resonance was called "Agape," and was a love beyond self and self-centered needs.

When I speak of Intuitive Mind, I am referring to the bandwidth of conscious that humans have access to that is in harmonious alignment with Heart Resonance. This means that we are functioning at a frequency that is absolutely present: fully here right now. If you have a thought that involves yesterday or tomorrow, you are not thinking with your Intuitive Mind. We are also functioning in a spatial domain that is also absolutely present; Intuitive Mind thinking doesn't take you away from where you are in your presence they way Survival and Intellectual Minds do.

Only Heart Resonance can fold space/time like this and keep you absolutely consumed with the singularity of presence. In this way, Intuitive Mind and Heart Resonance are harmonic corollaries. Where Heart Resonance is a coherent vibratory frequency in the quantum field, Intuitive Mind is Infinite Consciousness expressing itself through your human energy field and accessible through your specific bandwidth of awareness.

We are Infinite Consciousness knowing itself through our human experience.

I know that that's a big statement, and maybe a bit abstract, but it's a critical piece of the story.

If Mind does not equal Brain, then what does Mind "equal?"

So far, we can pretty much say that Mind, whether it is Survival, Intellectual, or Intuitive, is somewhat interspersed and equally distributed in the cells of our body. Whether you are still attached to the neuron/ gray-matter, brain-only illusion of this distribution or you are willing to extend that distribution of intelligence through to the DNA, there is some agreement that Mind has a root in the physical. I will venture to say that even the atoms not associated with DNA are carrier waves for consciousness (and there are lots of atoms in our bodies making up trillions of giant molecules: 2 x 1027 to be exact.) If you can take a breath and accept that every single atom inside of you is an energetically vibrating coherent quantum field, then take another breath and trust that that field carries not only information, but conscious and as such, contributes to your overall Mind.

For the past hundred years, science moved away from classical Newtonian physics, and thanks to Einstein and his contemporaries, it moved into an acceptance that matter and energy are interchangeable: a big step from the view that everything was just matter. Then the quantum physicists took that to another level, accepting that the idea of "quanta" or packets of energy actually describes everything in the universe. Along with this new viewpoint came experiments that proved it to be a very valid description of the world in which we live. One of the core concepts of quantum or particle physics is the idea of "entanglement." This is the beautiful idea that every atom, and the subatomic particles that make them up, is deeply entangled with every other atom in the universe. This means that what one atom is influenced by will at some level influence every other atom in the universe. Yes, the whole universe. Sure, the amplitude of influence is so tiny in most cases as to be inconsequential, yet experiments can show how directed influence, say upon the spin of an electron in one atom, can be made to occur in a totally different atom. The great thing about these experiments is that, 1) distance doesn't seem to alter how atoms influence each other; and 2) the resonance between changes in the two different atoms happens literally simultaneously: yes, faster than the supposed "limit" of the speed of light.

So here we are with the concept of folding space/time in Heart Resonance proven by the most hardcore, traditional scientists in experiments that have been replicated over and over again. I really love when our empowering and healing concepts get harder and harder to disprove…

If Intuitive Mind is guided by Heart Resonance, a fundamental function of quantum physics, then it's expression is in deep presence beyond spatial limits and infinitely entangled in the universal quantum field. The great thing about all this is that every one of us has and always has had access to this presence.

We all know this, but we assume that our Intuitive Mind (many time people refer only to "intuition" which is a small fraction of Intuitive Mind) is something that appears at random, or like a blessing in a time when we need to find our keys. Why do we believe this? Well, for one, typically our parents, teachers, spiritual leaders, etc. had no training as to how to access their own Intuitive Mind so how in the world could they teach you how to access it? We also live in a world that exalts the Survival Mind and the Intellectual Mind. Look how much of our societal reward system is set up to celebrate the good survivors (make a lot of money, raise your family well, etc.) and the great intellects (go to college, get a good job, etc.) Intuitive Mind simply gets relegated to the wayside, maybe pushed over to the artists, musicians, and poets. Look how much of the educational budget continually gets cuts for the arts… That's an indication of the cultural value of the Intuitive Mind.

The curious fact is, Heart Resonant Intuitive Mind is exactly what the world needs now more than ever. It's certainly what you need to help you navigate out of your Survival and Intellectual Mind dominance that got you into the corner you are in now. I think of the Survival and Intellectual Minds as bullies, pushy and domineering. They act the way recalcitrant teenagers do, single-minded in what they desire and clever in a manipulative way. These two Minds, actively operating in your consciousness (and subconsciousness) do their very best to bully the Intuitive Mind so as to get their way. The massive conditioning and cultural support they get which gives them their power is sadly centered mostly around fear. When we can learn to identify and activate our brilliant Intuitive Mind in such a way as to gently get these two "teenage bullies" to feel safe and then back down, our Heart Resonance rises in an amazing way. We start to truly understand what our life is like when we guide our choices and actions by our Intuitive Mind. To me, authentic Qigong practice is ideally suited to this as it activates the Qi Effect. Activating the Qi Effect empowers our Heart Qi vibration to make this energy familiar and applicable in very practical ways in our life.

Not only will operating from the Intuitive Mind bandwidth make the world a kinder, more empathetic place, but think about that quote I shared earlier, "You can't solve the problem with the thinking that created the problem." If all our world problems were created from the thinking of the Survival and Intellectual Mind, the only real solutions will come from the Intuitive Mind.

One thing that is clear to me. I've been doing my best my whole life to cultivate my Intuitive Mind, and it is clear that the systems in the world that like to control money, power, and politics will do whatever they can to keep people focused on their Survival Mind and Intellectual Mind because that is how humans are most easily controlled. Those brave and courageous souls who operate with a large percentage of their thinking and actions guided by their Intuitive Mind are the free thinkers and are sovereign in a deep way. They don't bend easily to outside or social influence, and they understand that their true nature is not only physical. They naturally intuit and grasp the Qi Effect and use it as much as they possibly can in every aspect of their life. They understand how their Intuitive Mind can hold the coherent image of a "healed" body and thus, they can be their own best healer. They understand how to rely on their Intuitive Mind to handle as much survival and intellectual tasks as they possibly can. Those who navigate life from their Intuitive Mind embrace the power of their Heart

Resonance to truly see each other as a mirror in some quantum entangled way, and this develops empathy and kindness and community.

Our physical "body temple" is spirit incarnate... you know this on the deepest level. Seeing Qigong as only an "energetic" practice (which many fall prey to) is a denial of the body requirement for full integration into the Wei Qi energy field. Of course it is integrated... our Intellectual Mind knows this, but the curious thing is that the Intellectual Mind cannot sense energy! Through its dualistic perspective, it only gives lip service to physical/energy connections and therefore can easily try and convince us it understands this connection, yet our Intellectual Mind denies the Intuitive Mind the ability to activate Qi in efficient ways. Hence, our body suffers while we THINK we are doing energy work like Qigong... It's fascinating, but true... and overcoming this changes everything for the better.

Giving in to our Survival Mind to care for our body has its own limitations because it cannot sense energy that well either. Its default is generally to pursue a quick fix approach that is very superficial and not sufficiently "deep." Depth, at the cellular, molecular, and atomic level of "body" requires subtle energy awareness and connection. Again, only the Intuitive Mind can access this. Survival Mind does a great job of convincing "us" that all is well and that we are on the right path, but it is ultimately subconscious sabotage that keeps us surviving and not thriving.

Understanding the Three Minds is key to seeing this interplay. The trick is to allow the Intuitive Mind more and more authority to dominate our processes. Dominate? Yes, from the Latin "domus" or "home"... like "dominion" or "domicile." Dominating our energetic process is to bring it home, to make it our home, core approach to what normally the Survival Mind attempts to hijack or the Intellectual Mind judges is not necessary.

I have been observing the way that the mainstream has embraced a trend toward "mindfulness" in the past 10 or so years. It's alluring to be drawn to this as so many are, feeling that they need to be more "mindful" and with that, their lives will be better in some way. I have spoken at mindfulness gatherings, and have talked with many who practice this, and I can only share what I've observed.

First, most all these people do not differentiate "Mind" as we have in this chapter. To them, "mind" is "mind." Because of this, I see their attempt to focus, manage, or empty all that they identify with "mind." To me, this is akin to "throwing the baby out with the bathwater," losing the precious gifts of the Intuitive Mind at the expense of the Survival and Intellectual Mind. I believe that without these clear delineations of Mind, we will forever be chasing our own tail and pointing blame for all our errant and disruptive thoughts at the whole of Mind. Why try to manage or empty your beautiful Intuitive Mind? It's like turning away the fire fighting crew who raced to your house when it was on fire! Your Intuitive Mind is your best resource and you don't want to try and quiet it along with the other two, sometimes troublesome, Minds.

Secondly, in the mindfulness groups I've worked with, they place gentle focus on the things around them. This can be a good way to build sensitivity to the world around you along with your relationship to them. The challenge here is that you are orienting yourself in a very materialistic/dualistic way, and life becomes the things and events around you. I guess for those who have a real challenge and adversarial relationship with their world, this sensitivity and appreciation may be a good thing. We have to be careful with this approach, though, as it can lead to a certain "overthinking" neurosis and a focus on duality with the world around them. I have seen this over and over again in people, including clients who come to me seeking a solution. Lastly, I don't notice a focus on Heart resonance in the mindfulness circles. It may be there, but without that being our primary alignment, there is a tendency to get trapped in a loop of forever managing the Survival and Intellectual Minds by using those very Survival and Intellectual Minds to do so. It's like the way the Food and Drug Administration (FDA) in the U.S. allows pharmaceutical drug companies to conduct their own efficacy tests on the drugs they manufacture! That's like asking a teenager to grade their own test! That just doesn't make sense as there will always be a tendency to benefit yourself. This is the same reason most Western therapeutic counseling doesn't work either, what therapist would want their client to "get better and stop paying?" The Survival and Intellectual Minds will always fight for dominance and manipulate situations to benefit themselves.

So how do we cultivate the Qi Effect and deepen access to our Intuitive Mind so we can end the madness within us? I believe Meditation and Qigong are pathways to this... Yoga and Tai Chi can be as well as long as they are taught from the more traditional and spiritual perspective and not just as a physical exercise. I've added a chapter to this book with some exercises that can help as well. The first step is to set your intention to choose this path of the Heart. Your Intuitive Mind is within you already, within every single cell, so do your best to trust this and resolve and transform any lingering inner conflicts, be courageous and make the choice. The next chapter will provide some deep insight into why that choice may be a challenge. Remember that even with the challenges that may arise, everything is possible when we move into Heart Resonance and allow our Intuitive Mind to lead the way.

Epigenetic Qi

I know that this book may already be making a fair number of Qigong practitioners feel conflicted, perhaps a bit frustrated, and probably quite concerned for my sanity. Even if you don't practice Qigong, you may have found yourself triggered by some of these Qi Effect concepts. This, of course, is a very good thing from my perspective. If everyone agrees with everything you say or do, someone in the group is not telling you the truth. Either that, or you were likely not acting fully from your Intuitive Mind and were attempting to make everyone happy... so you actually probably weren't telling the truth. In other words, you're not acting from your Heart. Heart embraces all yet isn't dependent on what others think, nor is it concerned about getting anyone's approval. In Heart Resonance, we are present, grounded, sovereign and free, and we really only seek what is best for the highest good of all.

Read on and see how all this weaves into Epigenetic Qi...

When we are find ourselves constantly making compromises in what we believe by always doing things to make others happy, at the expense of our own inner peace, we create a certain level of stress and inner conflict. Sometimes, this stress can become traumatic and lead to chronic, unresolved emotions such as anger, fear, worry, and anxiety. As the National Institutes of Health (NIH) in the United States shows in their many studies, a minimum of 70% of all illness and disease is stress-related. It is precisely this energetic imprint that effects us on an epigenetic, cellular level.

Epigenetics is a critical and emerging aspect of biology that clearly shows how mechanisms outside of the realm of genetics and DNA effect the development and actions of an organism. Before Epigenetics, it was believed that the genetic "code of life" dictated everything from our physical characteristics to how our body functions and makes proteins to grow and heal. We are now learning more and more about how a specific protein called histone exists in the environment surrounding the DNA, and picks up information from the energy around it. Through a process of acetylation, histone can heavily influence DNA. The implications of this is enormous since for the most part, DNA informs your body of what proteins it needs to make. Ultimately everything, every cell, organ and neuron, is made of proteins. To make this even more far-reaching, many studies have discovered that by increasing histone acetylation, we can improve memory access and actually rescue cognitive impairments. This means that what we think and how we think is not only affected by the energy that we carry in our cells, but what has been passed down to us epigenetically from our parents through our ancestral lineage also affects how we think and act.

Group Think, or "mainstream thinking," has become a widely used term during the few decades. Anyone alive during 2020 and 2021 realizes that we have entered an amplified version of human existence, and with that, an amplified version of human nature. As the author and spiritual teacher Ram Dass once said, "You're constantly running through a minefield of the perceptions of other people." When we meet our Edge, we act in ways that are outside of our comfort zone. Our Edge can be anything from the limits of our trust, the outer reaches of our belief system, and the limits of our ability to manage the processes of our Survival and Intellectual Mind. This is when emotions rise, when arguments occur, and when fear typically rears its ugly head. This generally happens when stress reaches noticeable and uncomfortable levels and our nervous system jumps into what's referred to as sympathetic dominance. In these moments of fight-or-flight, we either seek comfort in others, or sadly, attack them. This is a typical human nature expression, an intellectual coping mechanism, and an acquired survival skill. You can see how the Intellectual Mind attempts to dominate your thinking processes with coping mechanisms, and how the Survival Mind forces its version of survival skills into the mix to keep you from, well, losing your Mind. Group Think is what occurs when large numbers of people come to the Edge of losing their Mind. When that loss is experienced and survival is threatened, we can suspend our own thinking for Group Think.

You may say that this is an oversimplification and maybe even outlandish. Who in their right mind would give their power over to someone else… especially if it is an intangible "Group?" Well, track large scale behavior during the COVID Era and you may be surprised to see how individualized, clear thinking was very quickly shifted to a narrative that provided a type of comfort to many, albeit a false one. This narrative laid out a set of concepts (I won't call them "facts" because in many cases, they were absolutely not founded on any accepted science) and those concepts provided a tangible grounding to irrational, fear-based thinking. When we are in fear mode, as the story of a 'deadly virus' can so easily generate, we go into Survival and Intellectual Mind overload. When this type of sympathetic dominant thinking creates instability and anxiety, we reach out for any stable ideas and concepts that the Group agrees with that we feel will get us out of fear mode. Even if those concepts are not even provable or reliable, as long as they are accepted by the Group Think, we find comfort in "the Group." This is a tribal instinct, and is ancient within our Survival Mind.

After leaving the University of Colorado and my medical school scholarship there, I immersed in Eastern and energy healing studies with a couple of elder Master teachers for a few dedicated years. After that, I felt I needed to know more about the "mainstream world" and what made people do the things they did, which from my spiritually-minded perspective, seemed insane. So I signed up for several classes at George Washington University in Washington, D.C. During that time, I was studying with Barbara Marx Hubbard and running her non-profit as the Executive Director. While studying political science with some excellent professors who were all retired Senators with deep insight into the subject, I conducted a research project. In my research, I analyzed words and phrases from hundreds of television network news reports that I personally transcribed over the course of a few months. Remember that in the late 1970s, there was no personal computer yet to help with database analytics or even word processing for that matter, so everything I did was by hand and on paper. My professor thought I was nuts for taking on such a project alone, but he supported it and said he looked forward to what I would discover. My approach was to rate words and phrases spoken in all the newscasts from the four main networks at the time (yes, back then there were only four and no cable), and place them in one of categories: positive/empowering, neutral, and negative/fearful. I then looked for similarities in messaging. I had reviewed my metrics for rating these words and phrases with my professor so we had a clear sense of these three categories. I had large sheets of architectural paper where I created charts to manually plot out the data. It took most all of the semester to go through the newscast transcriptions and carefully select every key word or phrase. The data I showed in my paper was that far more negative/fearful words and phrases were used than positive/empowering or neutral ones. I also proved that many of the same phrases and precise messaging were repeated on all four networks. Looking back from the perspective of the COVID era as I write this, the exact same narrative script is repeated across nearly every mainstream media outlet and proves my original findings from 40 years earlier. Sadly, things have only gotten worse.

My professor was impressed that I completed my task but asked me, now that I was done, what I was really trying to prove. I actually couldn't believe what he said, and I replied that I wasn't attempting to "prove" anything, I simply wanted to see what the messaging emphasis from television news was to the unaware, trusting public of the United States. He shrugged his shoulders and made one of those "so what" faces, and he gave me an A as a grade for that class. That's when I dropped out of University for the second time, deciding I had a lot more to learn about what was allowing people to simply accept the disempowering, negative and fearful messages they willingly take in from the media on a daily basis.

At that time, I was fortunate to spend every day with Barbara Marx Hubbard and her circle of influential leaders. One of her dear friends Gene Roddenberry, the creator of Star Trek, and I had been having monthly meetings to discuss possible television show concepts. The one that we landed on together was the "Good News Network." It would be a channel devoted to empowering and uplifting stories about humanity. I remember how excited we all were to bring this to viewers, knowing that the world would embrace this type of messaging. We created a one-hour pilot episode, and I was part of the video and script crew for every shoot we did. Back then, a video camera weighed about 25 pounds and the separate 2" video tape recorder was about 50 pounds. After all this hard work of shooting and editing, Gene was satisfied that we had a professional pilot program. He expected the networks to be competing with each other to license the new television series.

Sadly, we got zero traction. Not a single television network even considered the series. Even with Gene, Barbara, and their many influential and wealthy friends in Washington, D.C., we couldn't get any of the networks to buy in. Curiously, the response from executives in each of the networks was the same. They said that their viewers won't watch anything that is always positive. Their viewers respond to fear. If we couldn't change the script to include more tragedy and stories that would scare people, they weren't interested.

I thought about my political science research project on cross-network positive/negative languaging and began to understand how conditioned the masses were to having their fear triggered. I realized how the masses came to expect and depend on this messaging to actually validate this deep, subconscious programming within themselves.

This is what sets up our epigenetic Qi environment on a cellular level and how our bodies interface with the Qi Effect.

I am bringing us back to Epigenetics because the energy of bio-psycho-social programming and conditioning holds the key to our individual freedom and personal transformation. I grew up in the 1960s and '70s when that whole industry went into overdrive. So many different people felt like they have the "key" to reaching "personal potential." I watched people jump from one workshop to another, from one "amazing" personal growth system to another. I was very curious when I was young because at first I thought I was missing something, that I wasn't "getting it" because most everyone I saw on that path was becoming more and more narcissistic and frankly, emotionally messed up. They would typically then make the leap to Eastern religions/philosophies in hopes that this would be the key. This cultural short-circuit, made by Westerners attempting to immerse themselves in a foreign belief system, isn't complete without including the contextual framework. Without the cultural conditioning from birth, something will certainly always be missing. Even when that conditioning is there for the people born into those particular cultures, those individuals rarely become fully empowered.

I've always enjoyed reading the Danish story that originally appeared in the periodical "Danmarksposten" 100 years ago because it captures so well how and why we believe in things. Danes are, of course, very proud of their Nobel Prize winning Niels Bohr. Bohr was a brilliant scientist in the 1920s and is considered one of the fathers of Quantum physics. The article states, "Above the door of his office hangs a horseshoe. The world-famous atomic expert was recently asked if he really believed that it brought him luck. 'No,' said Bohr, 'of course I don't believe it—but I've sometimes noticed that it works even when I don't believe in it!' " Oftentimes even when we don't "literally" believe in what we hear or what is thought to be true, we are like Professor Bohr and don't easily let go of the influence.

So how does Group Think and cultural conditioning fit into Epigenetics and the Qi Effect?

The fact is that Group Think and cultural conditioning are exactly what programs our epigenetic matrix at the cellular, DNA level. The specific way that our quantum field coherence becomes aligned and programmed in us defines in a large part how we behave and respond to the world around us in our everyday experiences. These behaviors and responses typically reinforce our shackles of epigenetic programming, and the cycle spins on and on. If you have children, you pass these shackles on to them.

"Genetics" defines genotype: your basic biological, gene-based characteristics that define everything from hair color to whether you have feet or fins. Phenotype, on the other hand, is how genetics work with your "external" environment to help you survive your environment in the best way. "Epigenetics" is a curiously different thing all together. Epigenetics is an internal environmental energetic that influences your cells and responds to external stimuli and can be carried around for generations. Epigenetics can influence a cell's gene expression to create a heritably stable phenotype without altering any DNA sequence. This internal environment is believed to be the "protein soup" in which your DNA lives. Your epigenetic soup is home to your genetic information. This "soup" is mostly a protein called histone that engulfs our DNA to both protecting and heavily influencing it through the aforementioned process, acetylation. The histone doesn't guide information directives to your genes, but acts more like the RAM memory of a computer by holding information in it's molecular and energetic atomic structure. Where does the data come from that is held in the RAM? It comes partially from your life experience and environment. The main influence is your parents, who inherited it from their parents. The data resonance within your histone soup goes back through the ancestral line, predominately along the female side. We will get into to the details of exactly what that "data" is soon…You may be wondering why the "female" side weighs in more heavily. Two factors determine that. First off, every human embryo starts off genetically "female," so the vibratory resonance for the ancestral mother-line is stronger. Secondly, though you may not realize it, we have lots of DNA: 16,569 base pairs comprising of 37 unique genes. Rather than living inside of our cell nucleus, this DNA actually resides inside of the mitochondria. Mitochondria are powerhouse energy factories that swim in every cell's cytoplasm. Our mitochondrial DNA only follows the mother lineage. Large-scale genetic research has been done since the 1970s to trace this specialized DNA data back in time and takes us to the very high probability of our "Universal Mother:" a Black woman on the African continent around 160,000 years ago. Yes, this is true for all of us and I love it. If we all could embrace this we would remember that all of humanity is truly a united planetary family…

In my pre-med classes, the Biology professors would proudly display a very organized and proper Watson-Cricke models showing DNA as a lovely and neatly arranged double-helix structure. Everyone cooed over it like it was someone you would be happy to have over for dinner to meet the family. The model was a large wooden contraption wheeled in by a teaching assistant who would stay busy for the entire class adjusting various spheres and dowels that had come loose. The professor would tap his pointer against the wooden thing, and everyone would nod as if they all fully understood exactly how a smaller version of this fit inside each of our cells, stayed put and functioned at 20%. Back then scientists were convinced that the structure of DNA was double-helixed, that DNA could never stray from that form, and that 80% of our genes were "junk."

Over the years it was discovered that if we stretched out this double-helix strand, it would reach nearly two meters in length. How in the world could something microscopic in size that fits neatly inside the nucleus of every cell be able to stretch out to almost six-feet? It turns out that DNA is not really a neatly arranged double helix, but is folded in amazing ways. It looks more like your earbud cord when you shove it into your pocket than a geometrically attractive spiral staircase. This DNA clump is wrapped up in an even more chaotic mess in the histone soup we just talked about. It also turns out that the 80% of our genetic code that supposedly does nothing and was labeled as "junk" is in fact a brilliantly engineered switching system that regulates the other 20% of genes by turning them off and on. You can see how the neat and organized picture of our DNA has eventually become turned inside out.

Our histone soup strategically holds our folded DNA in place, influences the genes, and most likely has influences and functions reaching beyond these two. The last chapter explored the relationship between energetic influences on DNA and gene expression, and we will continue with this concept in order to understand exactly how the histone soup becomes programmed and exerts influence over our genomes. There is a process called DNA methylation where a molecule called a methyl group attaches to DNA and, without touching or altering any genetic sequence, massively influences DNA relating to critical functions like aging and carcinogenesis. Added to all this is something called transgenerational epigenetic inheritance. As it sounds, transgenerational epigenetic inheritance is the science proving that epigenetic markers are passed down from parent to child. These epigenetic markers affect an offspring's traits without altering the primary structure of DNA. The fact is, each one of us has been given something that has been passed down for generations that is powerful enough to affect what traits we develop and express. This undoubtably proves that we carry intelligent, energetic fields within our molecular structures. This is why this chapter is so important to the Qi Effect.

As an example, gastric cancer is heavily influenced by epigenetic aberrations. Analysis shows that DNA methylation changes have a higher influence on gastric cancer than point mutations. We believed for so long that nearly everything about us was specifically programmed in our genes, and that "point mutations" in these gene strings were what created disease. Now we are realizing that there is something in the energy field of the cell that influences DNA that is responsible for the development of disease.

Histone is a protein that, like DNA, is made up of molecules. Molecules are made up of atoms. At each aforementioned level of structure, there are biochemical bonds holding everything together. Curiously, what makes biochemical bonds hold things together are the electrical charges and associated wave functions of the atoms involved, along with the arrangement of those atoms. "Electrical charges" are neither tangible nor physical in nature. To me, and many others, atoms seem to appear as "energetic waveforms" more so than physical structures. As forms of energy, they don't require physical touch to function and interact. Thing about a lighting bolt or WiFi signals. From all we are discovering, it would seem that our histone soup and even DNA itself are highly charged energetic fields. This line of reasoning leads us to see that, rather than biochemical interactions creating gene function, highly complex and information-packed quantum energy fields reside in the coherent and stable vibratory fields that we have been calling molecules. The way molecules combine to create more complex structures such as proteins and genes shows how these "information fields" store data and communicate with each other. This is direction of future of medicine and Quantum Biology that is accessible now for those who can understand the Qi Effect.

The way energetic fields are created, arranged, and transmitted is, in part, the science of electromagnetism. This very basic science is now well over 200 years old and is what helped my fellow Italian-American, Guglielmo Giovanni Maria Marconi, transmit the first radio waves over a distance. It helped both Nikola Tesla and Galileo Ferrara create the first alternating current electrical generators. This field of science is also guilty of creating multiple generations of humans bound to paying for cell data service and hunting for WiFi signals.

Now take that picture of electromagnetism and project it onto the histone soup surrounding your DNA. At the core of every cell inside your body is a nucleus, and in that nucleus is this histone soup carrying and sustaining an electrical field as it does it's job to protect your DNA. As an electromagnetic field, it by design carries and retains information. This "information" can be as simple as a positive or negative charge: right there you have two bits of "information." Yet, this histone soup-field is massive and interwoven with our DNA. As such, it has the very high probability of sustaining a vast amount of data. This is considered by many researchers who understand Quantum mechanics, such as Dr. Peitre Gariaev, to be a coherent quantum field of energy that absolutely carries and stores information. During Gariaev's work with Vladimir Poponin at the Russian Academy of Science in the mid-1990s, they published a paper in the peer-reviewed journal Nanobiology 1995 that pointed to the intelligence and information carried in a DNA molecule. In the experiment, they created a vacuum in a small, sealed glass container. They then inserted photons and resealed the vacuum. Photons are quanta of energy that we see as light, and they bounced around in the vacuum in a random and generally chaotic manner. This was to be expected: light bounces around until it is reflected or absorbed. Next, they took a sample of DNA and placed it in the glass container along with the photons, and then reset the vacuum seal. The photons that previously moved around chaotically appeared to assemble themselves into a coherent order. The photons assumed this ordered pattern in the presence of the DNA. It were as if they were either instructed to do so or were mirroring some energy. This sequence was repeated over and over, and each time, the photons went from chaotic and random movement while alone to assembling a coherent pattern in the presence of DNA. This surprised and pleased Gariaev and Poponin, guiding them to theories about what information is carried in the quantum field of DNA. During the process of repeating the experiment, photons were left in the vacuum after the DNA was removed from the container. What they observed seemed absolutely counterintuitive. The photons remained in their newfound, organized and coherent pattern while the DNA was not even directly influencing them. The only possible conclusion for how this was possible comes out of quantum mechanics. The field effect generated by everything in the field actually leaves an imprint on the field itself. This is why the "observer effect" is such a critical component of quantum physics experiments. Everything, every field and every thought, influences the outcome.

Max Planck, a German theoretical physicist, won the Nobel Prize in 1918 for his discovery of "energy quanta." His discovery essentially created Quanta Physics and moved science from a materialistic view of the world toward an energy-based perspective. The term "Quanta" is what we now know as a photon, the energy we see as light that was involved in the experiments by Gariaev and Poponin. It's no surprise that Planck's

Grandfather and Great-Grandfather were theology professors and that his father was a law professor. This is important because we can see that behind Planck's research and study was the implication of how the minutia of his work would affect both the world and human consciousness itself. He regarded consciousness as the fundamental building block of reality and felt that "matter" was in fact a derivation of consciousness itself. In 1944, Planck gave a speech in Florence, Italy called "The Nature of Matter." He made clear his deepest philosophical views by saying, "As a man who has devoted his whole life to the most clear headed science, to the study of matter, I can tell you as a result of my research about atoms this much: There is no matter as such. All matter originates and exists only by virtue of a force which brings the particle of an atom to vibration and holds this most minute solar system of the atom together. We must assume behind this force the existence of a conscious and intelligent spirit (geist). This spirit is the matrix of all matter." He went on to say that "Everything that we talk about, everything that we regard as existing, postulates consciousness."

At the time of Planck's speech World War II was raging, his home in Berlin had been completely decimated in an air raid, and his eldest son had been hung by the Nazi Gestapo. Years before at Berlin University, Albert Einstein had given Planck professorship and the two enjoyed played music together. Now, Einstein was being attacked by the Nazi's for his Jewish heritage. Planck resigned from several prestigious academic positions to show his supportive and humanitarian stance. Planck watched the war come to an end, passing away a few years later in 1947 surrounded by family at the age of 89. Planck is a hero to me, not because I agree with everything he believed, but because he never backed down from his friendships and political beliefs even in the face of massive Nazi, Group Think pressure. He is my hero because through it all, he managed to maintain a deep positivity about the power of consciousness and it's energetic role in our reality.

The emerging science of Epigenetics and Quantum Physics have a curious interweaving. There are theories on the ways memories, emotion, behavior, and the environment have influence on the cellular level thereby massively contributing to behavior and the choices a person makes. Quantum Physics supports that this is possible, and as a result so does Quantum Biology. If the mere presence of an observer can affect the outcome of a process at the quantum level, what is the influence of any thought or intention over our body and it's function? Moreover, when that thought or intention is amplified in intensity through trauma or extreme emotion, what influence does it exert over our body? If every cell in our body carries not only DNA but its associated histone protein "data storage" packaging, what are we carrying on a subconscious level that is influencing us without our awareness of it even being there?

This is essentially the core concept of Epigenetics. There is one more piece to it that is important. Our DNA and histone complex, along with our DNA methylation, respond to and store the energetic waveform state of what we are experiencing in our current life. These "epigenetic markers" exist within neural networks of the brain as longterm memories, and also have been found in the vicinity around DNA itself. Not only this, but both our DNA and our histone soup, along with our DNA methylation, carry the field effect of what is passed down to us from our parents and ancestors. Again, this isn't referring to the genetic information our mother and father pass on to us like hair color and other genotype traits. Epi means outside of, and so Epigenetic refers to the stuff outside of genetic information that is passed on to us. This stuff is much more subtle, and it carries the propensities we have for many of our emotional responses to life.

You may have heard of the research done by Japanese researcher Masuro Emoto on how thoughts and even the written word can affect water molecules. About 20 years ago, he carried out relatively simple experiments to show that placing a word like "love" printed on paper and taped to a vial of water would generate different shaped crystals in that water when frozen than another vial that had the word "hate" taped to it. People loved hearing about this and his book on the subject was a best seller. The basic concept was that if water could be affected by an external intention, then our bodies (which are made up of over 70% water) would also be affected in a similar way. To most of us in the energy healing world, this was common sense as we all recognized that even subtle external forces can influence us just as we are discovering now with Epigenetics. Emoto once visited Kaua'i and had dinner at my home. He had heard about my Watsu warm water healing pool where I offered hundreds of healing treatments all sorts of people from the musician Sting to local senior Hula instructors who paid me with a couple of fresh picked mangoes. I trust the power of water to respond to energy and intention, and my years of offering Watsu sessions to people who experienced transformative healing was proof positive. For people like me with direct empirical experience, Emoto's work was obvious. What was fascinating was that the scientific community did everything that they could to not only criticize Emoto's findings, but to actually slander him. Sadly, he passed away in 2014 and Wikipedia (which we can't fully trust on face value) still displays him as marginal. It's true that his scientific method was sketchy, but many continue to recognize how his research woke people up to not only the sensitive nature and importance of healthy water, but to how energy and intention can influence our bodies and the world around us.

In a more hard-core scientific approach, University of Washington Bioengineering Professor Gerald Pollack details amazing findings about water in his 2013 book, The Fourth Phase of Water. What Emoto showed in we'll say a more "intuitive" way, Professor Pollack scientifically shows the energetic nature of H2O and it's ability to respond to its environment and provide life-sustaining tools through its "fourth phase" beyond the first three we know as vapor, liquid, and solid. In this fourth, or liquid-crystalline-energetic phase, water displays a state that shows how it plays a much deeper role in processes like photosynthesis in plants or metabolism in humans, all in energetic ways that defy a simple materialistic, biochemical explanation.

To explore further how energy influences some of the most unexpected aspects of our lives, there are longitudinal studies that show how certain cultural propensities toward money and responses to financially-related situations are "passed down" from generation to generation even when a specific individual is neither taught these ways nor is the subject ever directly discussed. We all know certain characteristics that we have adopted from our parents just by being around them during childhood. That's obvious. What about the reaction you have to stressful situation occurring for the first time in your life? Something happens that you never encountered before, and then you find out from talking to your parent or grandparent that they had the same reaction when they were young. These are not just coincidences, these are examples of how intense and typically traumatic experiences in our lives create a quantum field energetic map in our bodies. As the Gariaev and Poponin experiment shows, we know that molecules in our body are coherent electromagnetic fields that can store a wealth of information and memory states. The emotional issues you have now that you blame on a traumatic childhood experience is most likely a drastic misinterpretation of the truth. You've attributed the wrong causal source. There is a very high probability that what you experienced as a child was actually an Epigenetic reaction from an ancestral trauma, an energetic resonance that was triggered in your innocent and unaware youth. We typically go through life blaming our child self or identifying with that hurt child. If we continue to believe that was the source of our trauma, we will never be able to heal. Until we travel down the Epigenetic highway and into our ancestral past, we won't be able to realize that we don't need to own the experience or the pain. It was simply passed down to us, so to speak, and it only appears to have originated in our childhood. Knowing this, we can free ourself from the false causality that led us to identify with or blame the child we once were. The same ripple that affected the innocent child continues to adulthood, but now, we can see it with the clear vision of Epigenetics. We can realize that we don't have to own the pain and can see it for what it is: an ancient energetic influence or trauma passed down from generation to generation. In that knowing, we can release ownership and release identification with it. We can see that there is no one to blame and therefore there is no victim. Going back far enough in your ancestral lineage you may even see that the specific emotion or trauma was tribal and not even associated with a specific individual. In that knowing we can embrace that some energetic sources have evolutionarily survival origins that have simply made their way into our subconscious so we can ground it and transform it. In that knowing we play our part in evolution and are free.

So, even though some of this epigenetic mapping originates from our parents, we can see that most of it was passed on to them from their parents, and many times farther back in our ancestral line. There is some good news in case you are getting depressed: not all of this epigenetic mapping is negatively affecting you. In order to make an energetic map that sustains over time, the internal experience needs to be intense in amplitude, and is why so many of the influences passed on epigenetically are of emotional-triggers originating from trauma. However, there are also epigenetic pass-alongs with positive components to them. These typically fall into the category of things that sustain survival. Facial recognition is one of the earliest brain developments we make as infants, and neurologically doesn't seem to be learned. Our bodies simply know and perhaps they even remember that this is an important survival skill. Other drives we have as children involve certain social skills which are rarely taught explicitly, we just know that playing and interacting with other kids is "what you do."

There are other ancient survival responses that can't be explained from being taught or learning from experience, they are "in" us epigenetically. These ancient responses include the fear of fire, loud noises, sabertooth tigers, and people from tribes we don't know. Isn't it fascinating to look at what we come into this world with before we even get conditioned by our parents, family, and society?

What is the most frustrating for the average person, is that they are being driven by these ancient subconscious triggers and responses even when the current situation doesn't warrant it. When was the last time you saw a sabertooth tiger? Many of our fear responses come from this Epigenetic mapping, and we aren't even aware that it's happening. Modern psychotherapy has no clue of these ancient Epigenetic programmings, so they will default to some random childhood experience of yours that looks similar to the "sabertooth tiger" attack and lock attention on it. If you think your issues all started in your childhood, you are missing the whole wisdom of Epigenetics and Quantum Biology. Learning to release your childhood experience with the willingness to go back into your ancestral lineage is what will free you. Your childhood experiences were simply the first opportunity your Epigenetic programming had a chance to express itself, that's all.

If Epigenetic research shows us anything, it is that we can actually shift these influences that hijack our lives and even do it ourselves. It has been shown that when we make these shifts, we can end the chronic trigger and response pattern. What's more, if you stop the madness, you reduce greatly the chance that you will pass it on to your offspring. This is big… but it asks a lot of you. What influences you epigenetically and sustains its influence is related to the people you associate with, the food you eat, the thoughts you carry, and generally the whole of your lifestyle choices. It is possible to make profound changes, but you have to realize how you got into the mess you are facing before making real decisions to shift things.

Everything around us is an energetic coherent quantum waveform and that electromagnetic aspects of consciousness are sustained by quantum tunneling into the Qi field and back. Our Mind has tremendous influence over the wave function we call our reality at micro and macro scales, and our thoughts are the one thing that we have absolutely any "control" over. Since this whole Universe is entangled in the quantum field, everything exerts some influence over everything else, and as such, every atom mirrors every other atom in some way. What we are experiencing is the dance of Qi and its relationship on our bodies and the world around us based on the extent that it is activated. This is the Qi Effect.

When we look at what I call Qi Epigenetics, we are observing in part the level at which Qi has been activated through your ancestral line. If the difference between "surviving" and "thriving" is based on a person's conscious or subconscious ability to activate the Qi Effect, then this component to your quantum field must be sustained in the coherent field effect you carry. Like all epigenetic core traits, this is passed down to your progeny. Some people have an innate ability to activate the Qi Effect. It makes sense that there have been people throughout history who didn't know anything about Qigong while inadvertently adhering to its principles. We know that the Qi Effect is enhanced through positive imaging, allowing Heart resonant to lead, and maintaining a healthy physical body through a high-vibration lifestyle. Look at various family lineages that sustain wealth, health, and power and ask yourself if there may have been something more at work than just good genes and financial resources.

In ancient China, Traditional Medicine was based on the Five Elements theory. It's important to understand this because Qi is part of this theory and will give you good insight into why the Chinese system is both brilliant and absolutely faulty. To the early Traditional Chinese Medicine (TCM) practitioners, and all those practicing today in any country, the Five Elements theory is the foundational backbone of clinical treatment as well as personal practice. There was no such person as a psychiatrist in ancient China. TCM doctors play this role, although they wouldn't use the same verbiage. Chinese are proud people, and even though women pretty much ran the show the men held the pride as the head of the house, ran the government, owned land, and carried the family name lineages. Let's take a look at a typical scenario I learned while living in Beijing that deepened my understanding of TCM. I was studying with one of the top TCM doctors in the country and lived at his clinic on the outskirts of the city. If you had to live anywhere in Beijing, this location up against the mountains in Badachu Gong Yuan was the best choice. TCM, in its brilliance, is a whole-person, whole-life healthcare system. While Western allopathic medicine basically looks at symptoms and then cross-checks the references for the best treatment protocols of the condition defined by those symptoms, TCM involves a sweet interaction between the patient and doctor that can last an hour. During that time, the doctor talks with the patient to find out what is going on in life at home and at work, all the while feeling for the dozen different pulses reflecting various organ systems, looking at the tongue for colors and textures, and assessing things along the way.

In this specific session, a wife brought in her husband. She was clearly troubled, and he was clearly the cause. The doctor was cordial with them, telling them where to sit as he gave me that momentary glance as if to say, "Here we go again." All the woman had to say was that beyond the norm of everyday life, there has been some excessive anger issues at home since her husband lost his job. The man nodded. That was all the doctor needed, he wrote some notes, got out some herbs, looked at the wife and said, "Your husband's Liver is out of balance." You could see both the husband and wife exhale at the same time as their shoulders dropped. They looked at each other and gave a slight nod. The doctor was once again a medical and cultural hero. He showed from his notes that the husband's Liver pulse was "slippery" and that his Liver Wood Qi was excessive while his Heart Fire was weak. This was obviously the problem, and by taking these certain herbs and practicing some Qigong, the Liver would tonify and all would be well. Both the husband and wife smiled and actually held hands for the first time, something you don't see much from middle-aged couples in China. They paid the doctor happily and left.

The doctor then described to me that it was clear the man's excessive anger issues, which most likely came from his job loss and his wife having to deal with him at home, had to be addressed. Getting into the depths of the psychology of the situation could get complicated. What all Chinese know, though, is that the emotion of anger is inextricably linked to the Liver. The doctor was wise enough not to deal with the complexities of the man's pride, and place all the blame on the man's Liver instead. In one fell swoop, the wife was happy, the man was off the culpability hook for any wrongdoing, he never had to be faced with dealing with his anger, and the pesky Liver issue would simply be addressed with herbs and Qigong exercise. I had to smile as it was truly brilliant theater. The patients walked away, problem solved. The doctor got paid and did his job well, both from a medical and a cultural perspective.

What this showed me, which I was starting to become quite clear on, was that TCM is all about "managing" a situation and not "transforming" a situation. Yes, patients are happy and yes, people move through their symptoms and feel better, but I never saw real transformation. People will argue with me about this, and that's great. They will say that the doctor got to the "core" of the problem and didn't just deal with the symptoms. Well, to me, this is just an issue of granularity. Sure, it's better to go deeper than just lessening symptoms. In that way, looking at the Liver issue is "better." The problem is, there are FOUR other organ systems and Elements involved in the Five Elements Theory, and it is an endless game of managing excesses and deficiencies to keep a person healthy. That's the brilliance of the system: it avoids looking at deep issues and maintains an ongoing patient/doctor relationship as the health management goes on and on. It is deeply faulty precisely because it doesn't involve transformation.

Until we can embrace a whole-person/whole-life healthcare process that is based on real and lasting transformation, we will be trapped by the principles of Epigenetics. Having the courage to know that we are influenced by our subconscious drives and then taking real and practical steps to be honest with ourselves to recognize them, access them, and use our Heart resonance to transform them will to be part of the Quantum Biology we will welcome in the next phase of human evolution if we make it that far.

It is always curious when our body messages us, reaches out in her "language" to discuss something. Another way of saying that is that our body typically communicates through discomfort, pain, and illness. This is the only language that our body knows we will listen to. Some of these "talks" our body has with our conscious mind are gentle whispers while some are loud exchanges. There is always something important to bring to the awareness table. On some occasions, our body is sharing what it is experiencing in relation to challenging and toxic influences and relationships in our environment. Most times, the source of these body communiques emerge from Epigenetic dialogue that has been submerged for a long time within us in what we refer to as our subconscious. Practices like Qigong, Meditation, Yoga, and Tai Chi are key ways to increase our sensitivity so we can become better communicators with our bodies and "hear" what she is saying while it is still a whisper.

The emotional expression that emerges from our subconscious holdings are what we seem to experience whenever we, and our epigenetic programming, are triggered in everyday life. For instance, when that "anger" bubbles up within you, it is best to welcome it into your Heart Resonance even though that may feel counter intuitive. Why would we want something "negative" brought into our Heart field? It is because your Heart is the power in the center of your torus-shaped Wei Qi energy field around your body, and this process is the true alchemical power of what we call centering. Instead of being "angry at the anger," welcome it into Heartspace with gratitude. The emotion, anger in this example, is simply the needle at the end of a thread that you can travel along far into the past, far beyond your childhood. Though we may be led to believe that our emotional challenges began in childhood, the fact is that was late in that trigger emotion journey. It was simply where you first noticed the emotion, the anger, express in a tangible way. Keep following the thread far back along the Epigenetic highway, past your parents and grandparents and beyond... and release causality in person or place as best as you can. Our challenge, and opportunity, is to travel back to the "essential Anger," the energetic source even beyond the first human to experience it. Getting to that point helps me remember that this emotion and feeling is not mine at all, and that I am simply resonating with an ancient vibration that I forgot I have the ability to transform with love... self love... Heart Resonance...

The challenge is that as we have learned through Qi Epigenetics, we are massively influenced by the energy imprinted upon us at the cellular level. We are also massively influenced by our conditioning and the world around from family to work. What we also need to recognize is that we are influenced by the very structure of our Universe. This may sound like I'm going out on a limb, but the concept of quantum entanglement shows how interrelated every atom is with every other atom. Yes, some influences are stronger than others, but experiments prove that once two atoms are entangled, they can influence each other even over vast distances. The concept of fractals in physics and mathematics shows how patterns on a minute scale influence the patterns on enormous scales, and vice verse.

Take note that we live in a Universe where nearly every spiral and elliptic galaxy is centered around a supermassive Black Hole, not the least of which is the one at the center of our own Milky Way galaxy. The Milky Way, known to the ancient Chinese as "Yin Hé" or "Silver River," is a spiral galaxy with hundreds of billions of stars similar to the Sun. Our solar system sits on the edge of one of the spiral "arms," and the reason that the Milky Way looks like a band across the sky is that from Earth's perspective, we are looking along the flat plane of the spiral as if we were standing near the edge of a round dinner plate. We can only see it along the flat surface and we can't see the actual spiral shape from our co-planar point of view. We know from observing other spiral galaxies, such as Andromeda 2.5 million light years away, that this circular, spinning spiral is what our Milky Way also looks like. Just like Andromeda and billions of other galaxies that astronomers have observed for years with the Hubble Space Telescope, and more recently with the Event Horizon Telescope (EHT), it is clear that each of these rotating, spiral galaxies are held together with a massive Black Hole at their core. We are realizing that there are more Black Holes in the Universe and even in our own galaxy than we could ever imagine. Just a few months ago from this moment in 2021 that I am writing this, the EHT team was able to capture the image of the Black Hole "shadow" in Messier 87, the supergiant elliptical galaxy known as Virgo A in the constellation of Virgo. By nature, a Black Hole can't be seen since it's extreme gravity literally bends space/time to the point that no matter or light can escape. Einstein predicted all of this in his General Theory of Relativity. Virgo A contains several trillion stars, and the enormous Black Hole holding them all together by its incredible gravity is over two billion times the mass of our own Sun.

Located around 27,000 light years away, the massive Black Hole in our own Milky Way is called Sagittarius A and is located in the Sagittarius constellation. It is "only" around 5 million times as massive as our Sun, yet it is compressed into a much smaller size than the Sun. This extreme high density creates an enormous gravitational field that holds together every single one of the 500 million stars that make up the Milky Way, including our Sun, and keeps them in a spiraling orbit around the Black Hole just as the Sun keeps the planets spinning in orbit around it. The challenge with Black Holes is that once they get started, they can't stop and their gravitational power draws in all available hydrogen clouds, gasses, and matter to use them for fuel. It doesn't stop there, we have evidence that our own Black Hole consumes whole stars on a regular basis. We know that Black Holes even consume photons, which means that light gets pulled into the Black Hole's event horizon never to return. We are learning now that our Milky Way Black hole is no different than others in the Universe, and that these supermassive Black Holes even eat smaller Black Holes.

Why am I talking about Black Holes in a chapter on Epigenetics? Hold on.

If we are constantly influenced by everything around us on both obvious and quantum levels, then we really need to look at our environment to see how we are being affected. We know what the effect of family or the workspace has on us, and we know what the effect of our country's legal and cultural influence is. Did you ever stop to think how the Black Hole-based structure of our Universe influences us? Every atom is entangled with every other atom to a certain extent, we know this to be true. We also know that every atom in us came from a dying star. More entanglement. So widen your lens and realize that we are living here on Earth in the incredibly massive influence of a supermassive Black Hole. It's not only that this Black Hole exists out there in the direction of Sagittarius at the center of our galaxy, but it's that this reflects the fundamental design of our Universe. In the fractal mapping of "large-mirrors-small," we have to take into consideration that the Black Hole Model of our Universe's architecture has an influence on how things are created on Earth.

How does this idea that supermassive structures like Black Holes are a requirement to hold a galaxy together relate to the idea that large corporations are running our world these days? How does the Black Hole Model reflect the move for larger and larger and even global, government ruling bodies controlling our lives? Could there be some relationship between the influence of the Black Hole Model and where healthcare seems to be going as smaller companies are consumed by larger, corporate medical groups?

There are no coincidences in a Universe that is quantum entangled.

Think about how after you stand around a campfire for hours, your clothes smell like smoke the next day. This is an obvious metaphor, but it still applies; You are influenced by the energies, actions and processes around you whether you noticed it happening or not.

The Black Hole Model of this Universe we live in is a powerfully influential force on your Epigenetic conditioning. How can it not be? Recognizing this should add a perspective to how you look at the many layers of influence that conditioned you and brought you to where you are right now. It's important to see how these mostly subconscious influences have pushed you to make decisions throughout your life. Influencers like the Black Hole Model vibrate a field function coherence throughout the world you experience. It has to be what influences humans with massive Survival Mind-based fears to acquire more and more wealth in order to manage that fear. This type of gravitational pull creates greed that can only be fed by more money and structures to support the acquisition of more. These structures we call corporations are fractal reflections of Black Holes.

Money, power and control all seem to go hand-in-hand, so this principle applies to anything related to them from governments to military.

Knowing this can help us clearly see what is going on around us. Then, we can use that clarity to look at both how we make personal choices, and how those personal choices may have been influenced by the Black Hole Model. You may not like to admit it, but all of the following examples appear to be influenced by the Black Hole Model: taking that corporate job because it felt like a safe choice, getting into a relationship with someone you don't really love and staying because they have money and provide security, and finding yourself stressed out because you feel driven to acquire more money or things. Even buying from large corporations instead of a small business can be a Pavlovian, knee-jerk reaction with influence from the Black Hole Model.

These energetics are mapped deep within us and into the whole global community. As we've learned from Qi Epigenetics, we have tremendous influence over transforming these subconscious programs by being honest with ourselves, choosing to make positive change, and focusing on Heart Resonance to engage the Intuitive Mind to make lasting and meaningful transformations at the emotional and energetic levels.

If we don't become individually sovereign and energetically "dense" and coherent, centered and grounded - like the Black Hole itself (and all that mirrors it) - we will be dominated by all entities that have that quality. It is not that we have fee compelled to compete by force, but rather, use 'wu wei' (effortless action) principles to enter into and energetic alignment within ourselves that allows us to be free yet sovereign amidst powerful forces that are part of the dense signature fabric of this dimension.

To the Taoists of ancient China, this journey was an individual one available to those who understood the Tao (the "Way") thereby embracing principles that allow them to live in a more natural way while understanding the underlying, available Qi energy. There was a counterforce at work in China at about the same time in history, Confucianism. Whereas Taoists followed their journey in a personal, individual way, Confucianists adhered to a strict set of rules and guidelines that defined how they should act in nearly every situation from birth to death. These conflicting philosophies emerged 2,600 years ago and eventually became woven together in the most curious of ways to become what the Chinese refer to as the "two pillars" of their culture and society. To reconcile these diametrically opposed world views shows the conflict that lies within China's very core of cultural psychology. This is not a judgement about any individual person; I have and love many close Chinese friends, many of whom are clear that they are Taoists. Why this is being shared in our chapter on Epigenetic Qi is because it's important to remember the massive influence acculturation has on us even without us even being aware. I was born into the Italian culture and trust me, I know the epigenetic influences that come with that across the spectrum.

I am obviously very aligned with the Taoist world view as I see this life journey as a very individual one. I have learned not to rebel against the "Confucianists" around me, but to simply understand how influences like the Black Hole Model and ancestral fear can drive a person to seek illusory safety in rules and an overarching "system." When I was younger, I believed that we needed to rebel and do all we can to "change the world." While at University studying pre-med, I had a part-time job working for Ralph Nader in his Public Interest Research Group. I was 18 years old and very motivated to take down the "evil corporations" and educate people on how to fight back again oppression. It was Mr. Nader who attended both Princeton and Harvard Universities, and took on Ford Motor Corporation to prove without a shadow of a doubt that one of their cars was dangerous and could kill people. He won the case and giant Ford had to take the car off the market. He also took on General Motors along with other corporations, and through his actions prompted some of the most influential changes in consumer rights and environmental safety ever to occur. The strides Nader took and their resulting changes to the system were part of what fed the enthusiasm of the 1970s.

This enthusiasm also led to a lot of what we call "New Age" attitudes that embrace the vision of global transformation, a world where everyone becomes "enlightened" and we move into the Aquarian Age. I would really love that to happen, and it would save me a lot of the time I spend writing books and teaching workshops. I know that what I'm about to share may not sound "positive," and you may feel that I'm not supporting the global vision of oneness, golden light, unicorns, and world peace… but in these many decades I've spent on this planet, I am quite clear that there will never be a "great awakening." This planet (I'll go as far as to say "this dimension") is beautifully designed by an incredible infinite consciousness to be exactly what it is. If there is an Aquarian Age, it is most likely one where people embrace this one-at-a-time, and by embracing it, gain massive transformational power.

If you can for a second, truly sense that there is a wisdom to the design of this Universe. Then, you must come to the conclusion that the way things "appear" in this material realm is just as it needs to be for our evolution. This evolutionary transformation is a choice: a personal choice. When we can see it, we'll understand that the ancestral epigenetic influences, the Black Hole Model, and even the sad atrocities we witness in the world are all Edges-of-our-trust: the trust of who we are at the core in our true, energetic nature. Each of these influences are triggers that can move us in two different vectors much like the Double-Slit Experiment that defines the principles of Quantum Physics. It is actually possible to move in both of these directions simultaneously.

One direction is to acquiesce and identify with the influences, which causes us to either become immersed in emotions such as fear or anger, or worse, try to fit in by compromising our truth and sovereignty. The other direction that these triggers can guide us is toward a deepening of our Trust in everything that defines us in relationship to the Qi Effect. Remember, "trust" in this sense is not a hopefulness about some future possibility, this Trust is a Heart-centered, very present knowing of our true nature. We can feel the "triggers" of the Black Hole Model, the "triggers" of our deep epigenetic conditioning, and even the "triggers" of sad things we see in the world around us, and realize that these do not reflect anything about us in our Heart Resonance. They are actually the antithesis of Heart Resonance. In acknowledging this, each Edge "trigger" carries a massive potential energy that allows us to activate the Qi Effect. Each time we activate Qi, we move from surviving to thriving. When we can allow this alchemy to take place in the Heart Qi field, we gain not only clarity, but we activate a certain transformation within us that energetically clears quantum entanglement with those very triggers. This is big, you will need to meditate on this and trust.

In the next chapter we talk about the Third Field. This may help you understand an efficient way to engage in the transformational alchemy of these triggers as it relates to relationships of all kinds.

What we can do right now is embrace the concept of Epigenetic Qi, and make the choices that we know we can make to begin shifting the chronic and habitual trigger/response patterns in our life by accessing the conditioning and programming that we have been subjected to. From there, we must do all we can to take action and activate the Qi Effect in our body/mind/spirit. Humans, by nature of our neurological design, are pattern generators. This is why we can so easily become "addicted" to everything from repetitive behaviors to drugs and alcohol. The only real and lasting way to stop unhealthy habitual behavior is to replace it with healthy habitual behavior. We can do all the positive thinking we'd like, but subconscious, epigenetic patterns have literally created neural pathways in our brain that are massive barriers to change. Healthy behaviors like Qigong, Yoga, Tai Chi, and to a lesser extent Meditation when done consistently, actually create new neural pathways and begin supplanting old habits with new ones. Use what we know to work and take advantage of our propensity for being habitual.

Techniques like NLP (Neuro Linguistic Programming) point to ways to be more specific and precise in "re-programming" ourselves with positive messaging and goal-setting. I understood and explored this path when I was a teenager. For some people it can be helpful. That's great. For me, I am understanding more and more that embracing techniques like Qigong can be even more useful in that they help dissolve our "programming" on a physical and energetic level and help us get into what people like to call the "Qi State." Researchers even use this term now, just as they do with "flow state." When we attain those states of mind/body/spirit, we naturally awaken our inner wisdom. You'll notice I transformed "state of mind" into states of mind/body/spirit because the flow/Qi state aligns all of who we are in those moments.

Qigong and Meditation help us cultivate our energetic sensitivity and interoceptive skills. Practicing "inner listening" to our body, we become active participants in not only our physiological health and homeostasis as we learn to positively influence the neural correlates of emotion. Instead of seeking the "Netflix Rush" by watching videos that dull our sensitivity, taking quiet time for yourself in a conscious healing practice could be a game-changer and life-saver.

This is the beauty of activating the Qi Effect: it supports us staying in Heart resonance and allows our Intuitive Mind to guide us. We are asked to embrace the incredible intelligence that we carry within us in the wave function of our quantum field, resonating in our DNA primarily, and most likely resonating the intelligence in every atom in every molecule in our body. In this way we realize that this "un-programmed" state (which we can call our "unconditioned" state) actually allows us to express the authentic nature of our sovereignty. With this comes confidence, inner peace, clarity, vibrant health, and Heart-centeredness all without setting them as "goals" or having to "program" them to happen. We realize that when we fully activate the Qi Effect, this is who we are and always have been. It's just been waiting for us to accept the truth of who we are.

When we notice epigenetic signs, typically played out as health symptoms or an emotional imbalance, it is time to take our personal practice into rejuvenation mode. This asks you to set an intention to "see" your challenged body system healed, whole, complete, and perfect. Rejuvenation mode also asks you for a daily practice of feeling how the "sensation" of Qi activating allows your challenged system to express itself in its prime design image, the "healed" state of your body stored in the vibration of your DNA intelligence. This is what Qi does. It is the life force that sustains and supports the intentional form and function of our body at the atomic-molecular-energetic DNA level.

We learned in a previous chapter about scientific exploration being done in stem cell research using electromagnetic energy in a way to positively affect protein dynamics, or protein-DNA interplay. This is a fundamental step in DNA remodeling and epigenetic control operated by a wide variety of transcription factors. This means that it is actually at the subtle energy level that we are influencing our bodies and even those powerful epigenetic influences that drive us at the subconscious level. To me this is absolutely empowering as it brings science, energy healing, and spirituality together and continues to show how we can use our latent mental abilities to activate Qi for our healing and transformation.

All my life I studied the brain in one way or another, and for many years I was CTO for a brainwave analytics company that I founded. It was based on a U.S. Patent that I was awarded for developing brainwave algorithms to identify states of Joy, Attention, and Inner Calm. With my partners, we developed a product that could show this in realtime on your computer screen. Many thousands of people used this and were amazed. Several school systems and large corporations also used this software to explore possibilities in the area of personal performance. This has always been my vision: to help people to learn how much insight our body, brain, and energy reveals if we only take the time to listen.

Ultimately our brain, and our whole body for that matter, is a energy field generator/transmitter as well as an antenna receiving the Universal energies dancing around us. Opening our Mind to new concepts helps to unravel epigenetic conditioning. Exercising our consciousness works the same way as exercising our body; keeping our "temple" healthy and in harmony allows the coherent energy field of our brain and body to embrace our potential and thus, experience new cognitive abilities and physiological functions. Having a healthy body that is stretched, fit and full of nutrients will allow it to function at a high level. In this state, we can perform physical tasks easily, experience high energy, and do things like hike mountains as part of that vibrancy. Our Mind is just the same in that respect, and when we can stay receptive to new ideas we build neural pathways that allow the "field generator" of our brain to support us in experiencing a totally new perspective of the world and Universe around us. Trust that we have all that is necessary to be able to discover our true nature and survive in this next phase of existence. The ones who understand this and can tap into their potential via the Qi Effect will be the ones who will have the integrity and strength to navigate through the coming challenges and emerge stronger in their sovereign power as leaders.

This Universe is perfectly orchestrated with all of its influencers and triggers to provide you access to the Qi Effect. This life-force energy is provided for your evolution and transformation beyond this dimension. Yes, we all live for a very short time in this particular dimension. That's the only thing we can absolutely be sure of. While here in this brief state of awareness, we truly are Infinite Consciousness knowing itself through our human experience and our human consciousness. Your unique sliver of that Infinite Consciousness expresses itself through you in a way that no other person can express. This is a gift and a blessing that we sometimes forget. Maybe our life here in this dimension is to remember our uniqueness as well as our deeply entangled connection to Infinite Consciousness who dances through us with every breath. In a practical, day-to-day way, our task is to build our core strength and grounding to sustain the ongoing transformation of our lives from simply surviving into actually thriving. There is NO influence stronger than that divine Truth within you. Peeling away ancient and current conditioning will reveal your Truth. Trust.

The Third Field: Qi and Relationships

Every person is in part defined by their own unique field of Qi-influenced energy. This is common sense even if you wouldn't describe it that way. We talk about the "kind" person, the "strong" person, the "weak" person, the "joyful" person, the "sad" person, etc. These are not just labels relating to moods or actions, these are expressions of their energy field. We simply don't think of things or people or even "moods" as energy as it's not in our modern vocabulary or cultural conditioning. This isn't just a Western limitation: in my years of living in China and all around Asia, it appears that the average, modern person has adopted a lexicon massively influenced by the Intellectual Mind that has been honed and developed by the materialist-based scientific revolution. This is a global phenomenon that has taken place over the past 500 years, and not a Western/Eastern bifurcation.

You can see what a challenge it was for many thinkers in ancient times to try and make sense of managing interpersonal relationships and discourse in ways that didn't rely on the sword or sheer force. The writings of 'Guiguzi' cover these topics, and came from the Warring States period of China when battles by war lords and their armies fighting for regional control were ripping the land apart. Farmers feared the harvest time when the warlords would move their armies through villages and take the food supplies they needed to feed their soldiers. To me, these writings have no "Heart" in their recommended processes of interpersonal engagement. They rely solely on debate skills, logic exercises, and cleverness. Lacking empathy, they ultimately focus on a scarcity mentality of I win and you lose. It provides good insight into the psychology of the Chinese culture and the thinking patterns adopted by China's modern leaders. The perspective of "limited energy" requires you to either acquire as much as you can or control as much as you can.

The ancient thinkers around 500 BCE from Greece to China saw life in much more energetic than materialistic terms. The Taoists of China called the field around a person the "Wei Qi" field. Everything you do, eat, think, and feel contributes to this energetic field. Your epigenetic, genetic, and even life karma contributes to this, so this energetic field, like every other energetic field from electromagnetic to to quantum, is in constant, dynamic flux due to changing influences. Traditional and Classical Chinese Medicine understands this field to a certain extent and both base their diagnosis and treatment on it. This is mainly done by observing the Jing Mai, or what we call energy Meridians, as well as other indicators ranging from your tongue to your eyes. Anyone who has had acupuncture knows that the practitioner will feel your various pulses to get a sense of how your various organ systems are functioning. This is a physical level indicator of our Wei Qi field, and the treatment uses carefully placed needles to affect your energy flow in order to balance and harmonize your current state of being. Energy healers such as Qigong Clinical practitioners may or may not be acupuncturists, but they will "read" your Wei Qi and focus on working with your Qi field directly. I will dive deeper into this topic in a later chapter, and you maybe surprised by what I have to say.

Everything you eat, think, get emotional about, inherit, wash with, brush with, and talk about will influence your Wei Qi field. Even the people you hang around with contribute to your Wei Qi Field. A relationship is defined by the energy exchange of two or more people. This could be as fleeting as a passing smile you share with a stranger to a long-term connection such you may have with your parents, spouse, or partner. In each of these relationships, a Third Field is generated by the intersection of "your" field and "their" field. This Third Field is a powerful energetic with it's own "personality" and qualities that are not only the amalgam of "yours" and "theirs," but will typically have its own unique characteristics as well. As you will come to see, I recommend that you treat all the Third

Fields in your life like a completely separate entity. Not you and not the other person, but a fully sovereign entity.

1+1 doesn't simply equal 2. If you've ever had an astrological Composite Chart calculated for you and another person, you will have gotten a glimpse of how 1+1 does not = 2. You find quickly that in the astrological model, which is just one way to describe the complex situation called life, this Composite Chart describing your "relationship" can have qualities and propensities that look very different than you and very different than the other person.

The Master teacher I studied with for years in the mid-'70s was, amongst other things, an expert astrologer. When I worked with this 81 year-old wizard to calculate the complex math required to analyze the geometric relationships between the planets, the Moon, the Sun, and our Astrological Houses, I had to refer to an encyclopedia-sized book called an Ephemeris. I lugged this book around because if my teacher wanted to create an astrological Chart, we had to consult the book in a moment's notice. My teacher would create Composite charts for two people, such as clients of his who may be having a personal or business relationship challenge. He would also create a Composite Chart for someone he himself may be considering starting a project with or doing an event together with. He also had a propensity for creating a Chart for the moment: for the exact minute, second, and location that an idea came to him or to us both in a conversation. This is called a Horary Chart. Consider this a "birth" chart for that new thought. The "idea/thought" itself carries a certain energetic vibration, and it was useful to see the quality and probabilitiesof that "birth" as reflected in the "Astrology Chart."

Energy healing and astrology simply point to probabilities. They are windows into what may be possible based on the concept that every atom in the Universe is entangled on the quantum level. It is for us to dance on this window ledge with an open Heart, listen, and respect the energetic influences that are present when situations occur, humans are born, or ideas come into being. It's all energy and it's all interrelated.

The Third Field is the dynamic interrelationship between two or more fields. It is not as "fixed" as a Composite Chart, but is dynamically in flux based on the myriad choices that each person in the relationship makes throughout every minute that unfolds. Nothing is stagnant and nothing is fixed in stone. Each person contributes to the Third Fields they are engaged in with every breath they take. Whatever you are doing to effect your own Wei Qi Field, you are simultaneously contributing to the Third Field of any relationship you are currently in.

You are most likely in a dozen or more "relationships" right now. "Impossible," you say. "If my partner ever found out I'd be in trouble, and that one relationship is more than I can handle already!" You know of course that your relationship with your partner/lover is just one type of relationship. Everyone has parents. Even if you have never seen or known them, you still have an energetic "Third Field" relationship with them. Most everyone has a friend or two and then acquaintances, clients, vendors, the lady at the market. You may not want to think of them as "relationships" but I promise you, they are. Each also shares a Third Field with you.

Think about how different would life be if we all could honor these relationships and their Third Fields for what they are. Each contributes to our well being, to the well being of the other person, and to the Third Field itself. Imagine being more Heart-centered in how you contribute to these Third Fields. What type of effect might that have on the world at large?

It is also important to known that these Third Fields never fully dissipate or go away ever. I love when people attempt to argue with me about this point. They tell me that they have fully forgotten about "that person," or they tell me how the effect of sleeping with someone only lasts for a week or two. There is also the argument that goes something like this,

"That person doesn't mean anything to me any more." You've got to smile. Third Fields never go away, sorry. Do all the energy clearing you want, trust me, you are only feeding that Third Field. I've shared about the massive influence our subconscious mind has on us. No matter how adept you are at engaging with yours and "resolving" issues, the Third Field remains. This is simply the nature of Quantum physics. Knowing that every interaction you have ever had on any level created a quantum flux, interference pattern of quantum entanglement that sustains in the vibratory quantum field. Relationships between people are fractal representations of relationships between atoms; quantum principles apply at all levels.

There is a famous and easily repeatable Quantum Physics experiment that "entangles" two atoms in close proximity so that their electron spin is the same. This is an indication that they are entangled. They then move one atom into another container, and place it on the other side of the laboratory. Next, the researchers change the electrical spin of one of the atoms and simultaneously, the atom across the lab changes its spin. What comes next is interesting too, because one of the researchers takes her container with one atom and drives it across town to another laboratory. She calls up the first researcher and lets him know that his atomic spin is still entangled with her. She's happy of course, for all the right reasons. Then, she uses a magnet and changes the spin of her atom and again, simultaneously, the other atom, in a contain miles away, changes its spin. This is one of the most basic physics experiments to prove quantum entanglement, and there are many more. All of them show that there is no apparent "time" it takes to communicate between the two entangled atoms. When one changes state, the other does instantaneously. Yes, "instantly" means faster than the speed of light.

It's just how things roll in this dimension we are currently in (if you are reading this book, most likely we share the same dimension.) Third Fields are entangled energetic wave functions. If one contributor to the field makes a shift on an emotional/energetic level, it will affect the other person contributing to the Third Field. If both people are tightly entangled, they could perpetuate old patterns forever. Maybe you've experienced this. Just like those two entangled atoms, a change to one will affect the other and vice verse.

I hear a lot of people talking about being kind to another person. I hear a lot of people talking about being frustrated with another person. I hear a lot of people talking about wanting another person to change and wishing that they would speak or act differently. I rarely hear people talking about their own contribution to that shared Third Field. This type of energetic responsibility never comes into play while consumed with what the "other" person is doing. We are programmed by our Survival Mind to see others as "different" or as "the enemy" or as "a threat" or as a "a tribal member." These are ancient programmings that lurk in the subconscious frequency bandwidth of the Survival Mind. Our Intellectual Mind also contributes to creating separation from others through judgements, prejudices, cultural norms, and generally limited life experience that lacks empathy.

Imagine if we stopped trying to change other people or for that matter, stopped even being concerned with what they thought. It sounds so obvious and simple-minded, but try it for a full day. I challenge you. It's a good exercise. Instead, put your focus and your Heart resonance on how you are contributing to the Third Field of each interpersonal relationship and interaction you have, and remove your focus from "the other person." Yes, this definitely extends to animals, trees, and seemingly inanimate objects. If you focus on your "spin" on the other person's "spin," you will simply get lost in the interlocked spinning. Rather, placing your intention on the Third Field you share takes the energy away from the entanglement (away from you and away from them) and towards your new shared intention. Try this and you may be very surprised at the results. You will be directing your Yi, your "bringing Qi to Mind" intention, to the quantum field effect that contains everything about you and the other person. This is much more effective in both healing relationships and sustaining empowering relationships.

The Third Field is real, and as much as it is dynamic and always morphing with your contribution (and the contribution of those you share it with), it also sustains its energetic influence long after you physically separate from the person you created it with.

If your wish is to improve a relationship, stop even thinking about the other person and place your Heart focus on the Third Field you share with them.

If you care to support another person who has a health challenge, stop placing your focus on them and "see" an image of them fully healed in the Third Field.

This is all somewhat counterintuitive, but put it to the test and surprise yourself at how simple it is to apply the principles of quantum physics that support the Qi Effect. To me, the only sustainable and supportive way that you can work/play with Third Fields is through Heart Resonance. Anything else will be in the realm of the Survival Mind or the Intellectual Mind.

Survival Mind will focus on compromises to make the relationship work, to help it (or you) "survive." Think of all the ways you are motivated by your Survival Mind. Your drive to survive pushes you to be with a good provider even though you are not in love. It keeps you in a job that you really don't like. These are the most obvious ways our Survival Mind controls our choices in relationships. There is also the subtle sense of "keeping the relationship alive," which is a curious survival drive that is deeply subconscious and arises from social conditioning. Think of how this emotional/energetic influence affects the Third Fields of your life.

Intellectual Mind is just as devious as it will "weigh and balance" your choices based on how good looking your partner is, their age, and what others may think about your choice for a partner. It will influence your judgement (and prejudices) about how smart the other person is and if you a good match on that level. All this goes for personal relationships as well as business relationships. I watch how people of all ages overthink their choices in the name of love and money.

You may want to go back to the chapter on Epigenetic Qi to remember the deeply conditioned influence within you that can cast a challenging cloud over your relationships. Resolving these ancestral programs will help clear your path to lovingly contribute to your Third Fields.

The only solution to this insanity is to call up the other bandwidth of your mind beyond Survival and Intellectual to reach your Intuitive Mind. It's the aspect of your Mind that remains when all the ancestral epigenetic and societal conditioning is allowed to rest. This is the abode of Heart Resonance. The ancients knew this as "Heart Mind" as they never even considered that the brain could handle all this thinking for us. They knew that the brain has a function because of what happens to motor and cognitive function loss after traumas to the head, but they recognized some deeper and far reaching awareness and consciousness that most likely resides in the Heart and Gut. Of course, as we evolve our knowledge with more and more research, we are finding out that they were correct. In fact, modern brain mapping techniques and the billions of dollars invested by the U.S. government alone in the past 10 years haven't revealed all that much into the mystery of our Mind as it relates to the brain.

To know the Intuitive Mind is to enter into Heart Resonance. You must know by now that when I capitalize the "H" in Heart, it's for a specific reason. This is my way of differentiating the heart organ in our chest from Heart Resonance, Heart Qi, and Heart Mind as the energetic aspect of Heart vibration. Intuitive Mind emerges from this place. This level of Heart is purely energetic/spiritual and resonates with Qi in a unique and high frequency way.

The concept of the sustaining influence of Third Fields after a "relationship" is complete is critical in our lives. For one, it should make us very discerning and sensitive about who we choose to engage with at all levels. Every person you spend any amount of time with will be contributing to a new Third Field that you now share and participate in. Sure, a short and fleeting interaction with the gas station cashier will have a high probability of not influencing your overall Wei Qi Field all that much. If you happened to become emotionally triggered during that brief interaction from a condescending glance that hurt you or an exchange of sweet smiles, this temporally short contact could have sustained a deeper Third Field influence due to the emotional component of the exchange. Think what a long-term relationship can do to a Third Field when emotions run rampant, left unresolved and submerged in the subconscious at the epigenetic level. Emotions are fields of energy, quantum interference patterns that have a coherency in proportion to their intensity. At a certain intensity, the energetic flux is sustained in physical form somewhere in your body. It takes on a resonance that sustains in the molecular structure of proteins for the most part. I cover this in depth the previous chapter, Epigenetic Qi. Suffice it to say, the subconscious is not some ethereal thought form. It has tangible, quantum energetic, and physical roots in your body. The resonance from this influences your Third Fields and every relationship you are or have been involved in.

Four Aspects of Relationships

It's useful to look at relationships when we talk about the Third Field, because as there are several aspects within any relationship. A relationship can range from business to intimacy, and can be with another person, animal, place, or thing. When we speak of "relationship" here, we are referring to any of those types of interactions. You may have a tendency to look at the following aspects of relationship as "stages of a relationship," notice how that line of thinking places a temporal component on your interaction while presupposing that you will go through some or all of them over time. The fact is, relationships are so complex, karmic, and reflect ancient Soul Thread weavings between you and others that even the most sensitive of us rarely see the full depth of any relationship. As we said earlier, Survival Mind and Intellectual Mind conditioning helps make a mess of most of our relationships by elbowing out our Intuitive Mind so that our Heart is only partially engaged.

Let's look at these four "aspects" of relationship and try to see each in light of Qi energetics and the presence of the Third Field. Some relationships may only exhibit one or two of these aspects and sadly, most relationships exhibit all at some point. We will explore why and how to avoid that as we go on.

Unconditional Love

Compromises and moving boundaries

Leaving and/or threatening to leave

Dysfunctional, with unresolved emotions that get you sick

If you are romantic, you may disagree with this whole concept. If you are bitter and hurt, you may disagree that love can ever be unconditional. If you are relationship adverse, you may agree completely because these aspects of relationship reveal how complex interpersonal reactions can be. Either way, this may be a good time to switch to a different chapter of this book if your palms are getting sweaty, especially when I remind you once again that everyone is in multiple relationships at various levels during every minute of life. These principles apply to every one equally.

Aspect One: Unconditional Love

To some of us, this is our deepest intention. Imagine if all of your relationships (business, intimate, and everything in between) were an expression of unconditional love. You may feel that this is an impossibility, and that is why there are three other aspects of relationships at your disposal. Yet, "unconditionality" is real and we have all had glimpses of this, even if we were unable to sustain it for long periods of time. This is the feeling you have, say, for an infant, where your love is beyond any need for a response. A love that consumes you and there are no boundaries to what you would do for that infant. Unconditional truly means "without condition" and that implies that no matter what the other person does, you remain in a loving space. I call this sensation Heart Resonance. Heart energetics activate the Qi Field in a uniquely harmonious way. The sense of everything being in alignment washes over us. Our perception is that we merge with the other in a unified way, a melding of oneness and natural entanglement. Our Third Field vibrates in a way that weaves us into a single fabric where thoughts and feelings are shared in sweet synchronicity. How could unconditional love be anything but the primary intention guiding all we do?

I have a bit to say about why it isn't… First, it's clear that most humans have a very strange view on the definition of "love." This is where people always want to jump in and define love to show me that in fact, they do know what love it. Most of the time it sounds like what I read on greeting cards or a post about puppies. Yes, love is a personal thing and who am I to say what love means to you. Regardless of what love means to you, there is an intention that is carried within that specific word. Anyone who knows me knows that I study not only Latin and Greek languages to understand etymological roots, but also how words and their energetic intention have evolved. Most times I discover how people use the most commonly spoken words in ways that have nothing to do with their core, foundational intention. That means that when that specific word came into usage, say 700 BCE in ancient Greece, people chose to use a very particular word to mean a very particular thing. This word then carried a deep intention and everyone who wrote or spoke it from that time on carried that energy with it. A word created 2,300 years ago faced lots of social, cultural, and religious evolution to make it into our vocabulary in the 21st Century. The intention that resonated with the creation of that word typically becomes conflicted with how we use it today. Love is very much one of those words that morphed over the millennia.

The original intention of love carried little or no emotion at all. The ancient Greeks had no less than eight words to describe "expressions" of love. Each was a condition or type of love expression. We still confuse these expressions with "love" in most every culture.

Agape: the ancient Greek word used in the Bible to translate the Aramaic word for love, describes universal, selfless, unconditional love expression

Philia: the affection we feel for friends, the name Philadelphia came from this

Storge: for family members and close kin, or even teammates

Pragma: the word "pragmatic" shares roots: it's a mature and practical, time-tested love

Philautia: the Greeks felt that this type of "self love" had to come first before you could love others

Ludus: when you feel playful, what we'd call "puppy love"

Eros: "erotic" comes from this passionate, procreative expression or love

Mania: the Greeks understood the destructive nature of obsessive, jealous feelings

What is at the root of love, though, besides these conditional states? From what I can tell, the core of love's intention is "where one places their attention/intention." When you think about it, what is the greatest gift you can give someone or something? Your Heart resonant attention. The only thing in life you really have any influence over is where you place your focus, time, and attention. At this level, there is no emotion attached, it is simply a choice of where you place your Yi, your ability to "bring Qi to Mind." Yes, it's curious to look at love that way, but my goal here is to show that at the essential level, love is a fundamental focus without initial emotional charge. It takes the Greek's eight words to define that "charge" and place it into an emotional space. It takes our conditioning to move love out of pure, consuming focus, and into the emotional roller coaster it can sometimes become. Conditioning. Conditions. Chaos.

To me, the complementary to love is when focused attention is aligned with fear. Even though the person or system carrying that vibration may not appear "fearful," they are in fact driven by that frequency of diffused focus and separation/disconnection at the Survival Mind level. This is why I feel that the wealthiest people are sometimes the most fearful. I have spent a fair bit of time with at least three billionaires and many other high net worth individuals over the years. Even though these people can appear confident and even like leaders, the more I discovered through personal interaction and sensitive observation was that they were absolutely driven by fear at their Survival Mind level. I don't place judgement at all, but I do recognize the force that drives them and their continued investment and business strategies. This survival drive is in complete alignment and coherence with the Black Hole Model that I have shared earlier. It is exemplified in all expressions of greed, consumption, and dominance. I don't believe in "evil" per se, but at its extreme, this type of "focused non-Heart resonant attention" is as close to what I would imagine evil to be.

Unconditional love is pure focus of Heart Resonance. What is more precious than that? It is certainly a challenge to feel this without emotion or conditions, but that is the beauty of this level of relationship. When we speak of Heart, it is not the emotional/physical heart (lower case "h") but in fact an energetic resonance of our Intuitive Mind that has none of the charge of Survival Mind or Intellectual Mind. Heart Resonance isn't thinking based on judgement and it doesn't know about past or future; is exists in the singularity of presence.

This sounds like some unattainable fantasy, but we've all had tastes of it. To me, Qigong and meditation practice are the pathway to sustain Heart Resonance at the Intuitive Mind level so that it activates the Qi Effect and can become more and more accessible in all we do including becoming the primary influence over our Third Fields. Imagine if our primary intention was to feed our Third Field with Heart Resonance. When this becomes your primary contribution to relationships, everything shifts in amazing ways. And when you can't sustain that, you move to the second aspect of relationships...

Aspect Two: Compromises and moving boundaries

There is a general perception amongst many people who come to me for consultation that all relationships require compromise and boundaries, both of which are in a constant state of adjustment. We have been conditioned to believe that compromising your wishes, your integrity, and your dreams are all part of maintaining a "healthy" and sustainable relationship. I have to agree. If you want a relation that is based on compromise and boundaries, then yes, you have just defined what is required. This is most definitely an aspect of relationship that many confront every day. Think about how you "pick your battles" and make compromises to get what you want or to have a situation go a certain way. Think about how you compromise what you believe im to avoid conflict. Think about how you compromise your dreams to keep a high-maintenance partner from going off the deep end. Compromise is a management tool used in most relationships from marriages and partnerships to workplace and commerce. Compromise takes a lot of energy as we are always consciously or subconsciously adjusting and regulating the various factors involved in our compromises. It's no surprise that people are exhausted in relationships, and it's why pent-up and unresolved emotions from managing our compromises rise up at times to overwhelm and disrupt us.

Boundaries are also another management tool in relationships that we create consciously or inadvertently. I even hear people talk about "healthy boundaries" and I suppose in relationships that are pure business, this may be a practical matter. Sadly, even in loving/intimate relationships, people create a massive network of boundaries typically fed by fear. These boundaries, by definition, reduce our ability to connect with another person and they keep others at a distance from us. Think how this affects our Third Field. You might say that they are necessary. If they serve you, then it's your choice. But it's important to be conscious of how boundaries impact your Wei Qi Field and how that contributes to the Third Field you share with the other person, especially if it is an intimate relationship. When we look at relationships energetically and try and visualize the boundaries we sustain, it's no doubt another energy/time suck on our being. Every choice we make effects our energy field, and a times comes to ask why we make certain choices.

Some people have the perception that it takes much more energy to deal with a dysfunctional relationship, and that it takes "less energy" to compromise, so they live a life of compromises and moving their boundaries all the time. They usually think any of this takes less energy and is less draining and less stressful than actually leaving the relationship… which leads us on to the next aspect.

Aspect Three: Leaving and/or threatening to leave

Yes, this is an aspect of relationships because if you think about what you observe in the world, many relationships sustain for inordinate amounts of time in the state of transitioning out of that very relationship. How many people do you know who talk about leaving their job or leaving their spouse or partner, yet continue on in the relationship? I have seen people stay in that state for years. Some people actually physically leave the relationship and move out for a while only to return. Others leave emotionally and return for a while, and then leave again. So it is quite clear that an aspect of many relationships lies in the tumultuous state of chaos, the push/pull of wanting to leave, threatening to leave, or actually moving on. A relationship's Third Field doesn't go away when you walk out the physical or emotional door: It sustains whether you like it or not.

Leaving a relationship, whether you instigated it or not, is a complex energetic state woven with stress, emotion, Survival Mind triggers, and epigenetic activation. It can be destructive to our state of mind, our spirit, and our health.

As I continue to remind, the National Institutes of Health in Washington, D.C. cites in their studies that stress is the cause of 70% of most all disease and illness. Most of us have a "stress-aversion" tendency that is a coping skill and a basic survival mechanism within us. It typically converts to the "Compromise/Boundaries" aspect of relationships.

If you are this type of person, you may be able to relate to the above relationship example. You have defined how much "energy" it takes to move through a relationship, and you take the most efficient path. Of course love comes into play, and you may say that with love, compromise and moving boundaries are just part of it. We can see how these two different perspectives on how much energy it takes to maintain a healthy relationship can play out in normal life. As long as energy feels like a limited commodity, we will make insane choices. "Insane" comes from the Latin root "in" not + "sanus" healthy. How often do we make unhealthy choices when it comes to relationships on any level?

Aspect Four: Dysfunctional, with unresolved emotions that get you sick

There are also people that will not compromise much or move their boundaries very far. They feel like all of that takes "too much energy" and is the other person's responsibility as it is "the other person's fault." When challenges in a relationship occur, they will vacillate between "threatening to leave" or go directly to the dysfunctional mode which avoids dealing with unresolved issues. Many times these people get emotionally or even physically sick in the process.

Deep ancestral Epigenetics are typically massive influencers on the subconscious level. Soul Thread weavings of both parties create many karmic Edges and challenging triggers, and although they can have massive potential for healing and transformation if people move into Heart Resonance, they sadly play out in co-dependent situations and even spousal abuse that turns chronic. Even in relationships that can carry the appearance of being "socially acceptable" from intimate to business, a deep level of dysfunction can be taking place as one or both parties puts out a massive amount of energy/emotion to sustain the dysfunction at acceptable levels.

Using these four simple definitions for your relationships can be very helpful. Yes, you can add many more levels, but it's a useful exercise to be minimal. In this way, our Intellectual Mind can rest and we can feel more deeply with our Intuitive Mind. These relationship aspects are not a scale, and are not judgemental; everyone is where there are in the myriad relationships that they are currently in or have been in. Each aspect of relationship has equal potential for being sustainable. In other words, people can stay in a job relationship or a love relationship for years or even a lifetime and not shift out of a single type of relationship.

My paternal Grandmother sustained Unconditional Loving relationships with everyone in our family her whole life. It's amazing to say that or even think it was possible, but it's true and anyone in my family who knew our Nonna Carmella Angelli would agree. Some souls are like that and have an incredible way of immersing in Intuitive Mind through Heart Resonance. Because of my Nonna, I have always felt that this state was possible in human consciousness and in human relationships.

As I was becoming the eldest of nine children, my parents were busy being pregnant and so they would leave me with Nonna. Of course as a two year-old, the sensation of being held by your grandmother who sung to you in Italian and fed you from her garden was exquisite. I remember times when she and I would be laughing and then my parents would drive back to fetch me. I would instantly act like I was sleeping in my Nonna's lap so that when my parents walked over she would tell them to leave since I was napping and they could come back later. Grandmother knew that I really didn't want to head back to the parental chaos and would rather revel in the sweet resonance of unconditional love.

This wasn't the only reason I know Nonna was a soul capable of unconditional love. As I got older, I watched every Sunday as my family would join with the families of four other sons of Nonna at her home. There were another two Uncles who never married and an Aunt who hadn't yet married, and since those three lived with Nonna they joined together at the big table for the weekly gathering. Food was plentiful and seasonal, and with so many people these gatherings were too large for eating a main meal. They were more focused on espresso and desserts. Nonna would sit at the head of the table, nearest the stove. The Aunt who lived with her sat to her right, and all the daughters-in-law sat on that side of the table in pecking order based on age. On the other side of the table were the men: the Uncles who lived with her sat closest to Nonna and the other Uncles sat next to them. I didn't learn of unconditional love from anyone but Nonna. When the inevitable Italian temper would rise (these gatherings were therapy sessions for the most part) Nonna would point her crooked, arthritis-ridden finger at the person getting out of hand and say something like, "No, no... amore, prego..." This little wizard less than five-feet tall commanded the room and everything regained a momentary calm silence. Someone would inevitably break the silence and ask if anyone wanted an espresso as the family got back to the matters at hand.

Once in a while, someone (usually one of the Aunts) would get emotional around the table. Imagine all of the grandchildren standing in a ring behind the sitting Uncles and Aunts watching this theater. Only the youngest would be playing in the other room: the rest of us wouldn't miss this performance for a minute. When the Aunt would talk about the terrible situation she was facing in her family and that there was no obvious solution, everyone shouted out their way to fix the situation and none of them were close to a reasonable answer. There was really only one way to resolve things, and Nonna knew how. First, she would tell her daughter sitting next to her to make the Aunt in question a cup of espresso. She did and the Aunt drank it. Then Nonna would get up and walk around the table to the Aunt and whisper to her, "La tazza." (bring the cup.)

They would then sit next to each other in the dining room (still within earshot of the curious group) and Nonna would ask my Aunt a couple of key questions and wait for the answers. Nonna would then take the espresso cup and look into the grinds sitting at the bottom. There was this amazing moment of quiet where I'm sure no one was breathing. Then, with ease and grace and in the most non-judgmental voice, Nonna would lay out exactly what the problem was saying, "Guarda, guarda" (look, look) gesturing to the grinds in the cup. From them to her it was clear, and because the solution was "in the grinds" it was no longer a personal opinion. Nonna didn't know about quantum physics entanglement, but she was a master of it. She would go on to explain the solution, stating in no uncertain terms what needed to be done based on the message laid out in the pattern of the coffee grinds. There was never a retort from any Aunt in all the sessions that I witnessed. What Nonna channeled was beyond opinion: it was a reflection of wisdom itself.

This may be what we call unconditional love.

We do live in a world that is quite complex with many influencers and stressful conditions. Unconditionality is a challenge, so we embrace compromise and boundaries. For most, this is the only practical solution to surviving in a world that is comprised of relationships between people that are not always Heart-centered. In fact, most people tell me that this is normal, so I will accept that.

The two most important things about compromise and boundaries in a relationship is that it is best if they are as transparent as possible and that both (all) parties agree to them. Only when compromise and boundaries become unspoken and one-sided do movements toward other dysfunctional aspects of relationship start to occur. Transparency doesn't necessarily mean that you need to always talk about every little compromise, but there are ways to keep the dynamic process open and clear. This can lead to healthy and empowering relationships.

Besides what you directly share with your relationship partner, remember about the Third Field. I can't emphasize enough about the value and importance this energetic quantum field effect is in light of the Qi Effect.

Imagine a garden that you and someone you are in relationship with created. Each of you dug in the earth, cleared the weeds, chose the flowers to buy, and then planted them together. This is your mutual creation. It's a simple way to look at the Third Field that you both share.

When you are both far from the garden, the flowers continue to grow just as the Third Field sustains whether you are there or not. If you stay away from the garden too long and it doesn't rain enough, the flowers will get stressed. If you stay away longer, weeds will start to intrude and begin to rob the flowers of nutrients they need. This can also be a metaphor for the Third Field. Neither you nor your partner have come near the garden, yet its evolution continues regardless. No matter what you or your parter may be doing to yourself or feeling about yourself, or thinking or feeling about the other person, there is no energy being contributed to the neglected garden itself.

One of you then chooses to return to the garden, and seeing how dry it is, you water the flowers and they respond in a positive way. The other one also chooses to go to the garden on another day and upon seeing all the weeds, begins removing these pesky intruders to give the flowers breathing space. Until one or both of you made the choice to place your intention on the garden (the Third Field), the energetic condition there remains an unloved mess.

The Third field is critical for healing practitioners to understand. Remove thoughts of your clients and patients and of their bodies, and instead, radiate Heart resonance to the field you share with them. Embrace their essence and Qi field with love… see them healed and strong. This energy will support them best. Shift your thought from their limited and challenged bodies and align your focus and awareness in the Third Field, which carries the image of their whole and complete, fully healed essence. Obviously, your whole and complete, fully healed essence resides in that space as well, so healers who understand this can only be energized and contribute to their own healing in the process of their healing energy work with others. I have observed over the decades that healers who get exhausted after their treatments are focused only on their patient/client and not on the Third Field. They may even tell me that they were working on their energy body, but still, this is not the Third Field. When your patient/client's body or even energy field is your focus, you are still operating in duality, and this goes back to our Container-vs-Conduit discussion in the chapter "Meet the Qi Effect." Many healers appear effective even when working under their limiting beliefs, but I've noticed that most healing effects are short term because of it. Until the Third Field is addressed and harmonized, your relationship energetic limitations will linger and healing will typically be symptom-calming and not fully healing or transformative. Even if a healer only works on a patient/client once, the Third Field has been culled into existence. Understanding that what I am sharing here is a massive belief-system shift and engaging in the Third Field during healing sessions will reap amazing benefits that will be long-lasting and life-changing.

Just as we have these Third Field energetic dynamics between two people, of course these field dynamics apply to groups equally. There is also what we can refer to as the Global Third Field. We all know this sensation when we feel for the Earth and everyone on it. The Buddhists always pray for "all sentient beings" as it is part of that philosophy and practice to be inclusive and Heart-centered. Praying for every one of the 7.9 billion people on this planet is daunting and impossible to include everyone unless in very loose terms. Understanding the Global Third Field shifts the focus from all the individuals in the world, and instead radiates your Heart resonance to the single shared Third Field of the planet. In this way, you contribute something meaningful to the quantum field, your coherent Yi focus of love. Even though we can't help everyone that we may like, we can radiate our Heart resonance into the vast entanglement and trust we are doing our part.

Going out a bit wider beyond a human-focus, the concept of Divine 'love' could then be considered the "attention" of Infinite Consciousness of the Creator which influences and feeds the creation process itself and all that is created. What the ancient Chinese Taoists refer to as Yuan Qi, or the "primordial life-force" that emerges from the Wuji emptiness to start the creation process carries this Divine love to the process of creation, birth, and all that is created and born.

Our relationship with Qi also has it's own third field, and it seems to take the form of our apparent physical body. This is the deepest essence of the Qi Effect. It may seem strange to think of it that way, as third fields between people are solely energetic fields. It is only our perspective that the body is in fact "physical." For practical purposes, it is. But energetically it is a coherent quantum wave function and takes on a "third field" role between our consciousness and Qi. Feel into this again: our body itself is the manifestation of the Third Field between our consciousness and Qi. It is the most important relationship we have in this Dreaming we call life…

This is the essence of the Third Field: the energetic field effect of quantum entanglement that you share with virtually every person you have encountered to one extent or another. This is what vibrates within every single relationship. Of course, there are practical and obvious things to do to keep relationships healthy, empowered and vibrant such as communicating clearly, listening deeply, loving touch, the occasional gift, etc. These are obvious, and my task is not to state the obvious, but to inspire the subtle within you that dances at the Qi level. When we learn to "tend our gardens" energetically, stop pointing Survival and Intellectual Mind "fingers," and stop being so concerned with what the "other" person is doing, we may be surprised at how simple applying the Qi Effect to relationships really is.

"A reciprocal relationship enables a qualitative relation between structure and background, in which each has the potential not only to "impact" the other, but to generate transformations in the nature of what each actually is... More broadly considered, the notion of reciprocal relation allows for nested, mutual influence even between macroscopic processes and those at the atomic level, indicating the complexity of the pathways through which the qualitative infinity of nature may manifest."

"The Essential David Bohm" edited by Lee Nichol

Qi Curiosities

During my 25 years of living and traveling annually in China and bringing large groups there to study Qigong and Traditional and Classical Chinese Medicine, I got to spend quality time with amazing elder Masters of the Taoist and Buddhist tradition. I also got exposed to many things that were on the fringes, and some that defy logic.

My intention in this chapter is not to tell stories that take you into the realm of those fringes because I don't feel they are ultimately empowering or practical. That said, it is good to know a little bit about some of these aspects that relate to Qi so that you can make your own mind up about how you'd like to incorporate the Qi Effect into your life. It is my personal view that the most amazing expressions of the Qi Effect have much more to do with helping us discover a practical way to thrive and live a peaceful and healthy life than they do with displays of extraordinary feats. Living a joyful, grounded, vibrant life is really about the most extraordinary thing anyone can do these days!

When I was living in Beijing and studying Qigong, martial arts, and TCM with with various Lao Shi (old teacher) such as Master Duan Zhi Liang, there was a traditional way to study with an elder wizard. You basically devoted 24 hours of your day for as long as they were willing to engage in spending time with you. This meant everything from doing Qigong practice in the park together at dawn to assisting in patient treatments, eating meals together, and going on spontaneous adventures which you were rarely told any details about; you just got on a bus or jumped into the back of a truck and went. One of these adventures with

Master Duan was to a downtown conference center. This was about the antithesis of anything Duan-like. Though he lived in Beijing city proper, his apartment was next to the Bai Yun Guan (White Cloud Temple) with amazing Taoist temple grounds and the nearby river to soften the energy of this massive metropolis. I followed Master Duan as we made the many bus connections and weaved through traffic to our destination. I can see it all now, Duan at 95 years-old with a long grey beard in his white, flowing Taoist garb and black Chinese slippers. Me, barely 30, carrying the 10-point deer antlers he liked to have with us, a couple of swords in sheaths, and a white cloth bag filled with herbs and who knows what else. We finally show up at the convention center and it is quite busy. The guards at the door seem to be being very particular about who they let into this convention. I watched several arguments and many people got turned away. Master Duan walks right past the long line of people waiting to get in (I was used to this with him) and he says something to the guards. They open the door and usher me and the elder Master inside. Of course I'm still trying to make sense of what all this was about and why we were there when we gaze out into a very large hall with a stage at one end filled with people, seats in the main area, and various displays all around the perimeter.

Duan gestures to the stage and shook his head. He says that most of these people were "bu hao" (not good), but I was used to this by now as he was a wonderful old curmudgeon and very discerning with sharp opinions about nearly everything. I figure he's earned it at 95. One of the on-stage Masters he did like was Professor Fang Li Da, who was also the only woman. She was the Director of China's Medical Research Institute who did very thorough work on how Qigong can effectively work to cure cancer. He introduced me to her and she was very respectful to him. I got to meet her another time in Beijing and years later, again in San Francisco in 1997 when I taught a class at Effie Chow's second World Congress on Qigong (the same Congress that I had helped her put together years before.)

Master Duan had also earned respect from many, many people, and I had never experienced this side of him before in the daily, casual experience with him I enjoyed. As I walked behind him at the packed conference and we made our way through the hall, nearly every person we encountered in the crowd addressed him by name "Duan Lao Shi" (a very respectful way to say "Elder Teacher Duan.") He usually just nodded and with only a few of the elders he met along the way did he smile and say something that made them both laugh. As we walked, we passed display after display and I was starting to catch on to what we were attending. It was a Qigong Master Convention. Imagine hundreds of attendees and it turned out only qualified (and CCP government-registered) Qigong Masters could attend. Now I knew why the guards at the door were so adamant about who came in. Each display had some Qigong Master standing next to it talking to whoever would listen about what Qigong service he or she offered, of course discussing their going rate. Many offered healing services, with some practitioners talking about how much they charged "per body part" they healed. Many said that they wouldn't charge unless they actually healed someone, which I thought was novel. I later discovered that that was the ancient Taoist way of any respectable doctor. Another display had "before-and-after" photographs of rice paddies or farmland. The Qigong Master explained that, for a very reasonable fee, he would come to your freshly planted crop and perform some Qi energy work on your plants to help them grow. Another display I remember had some metallic device that reminded me of an old-fashioned TV antenna like the ones we had on our television set at kids. The Qigong Master was explaining how she could place medicinal herbs in the little compartment in the middle of the antenna and then radiate her Qi through the device and toward a person far away. All these conversations were quite matter of fact, as if you were at a plumber's convention and salespeople were talking about pipe fittings.

I have so many other personal experiences that I can share about Qigong Masters all over China sharing their "take" on how they can manipulate Qi. Once, to meet up with a particular Qigong Master who was very impressed by overt displays of supposed Qi manipulation, I traveled far to the south eastern area of China to meet her. She wanted me to see this Qigong Master who could stop a clock. What could I say? Every time I thought I had seen everything in China, I was proven wrong; there was always another curiosity waiting in the next village it seemed. Imagine this skinny, middle-aged chap sitting at a table with a clock on the wall in this nondescript room. He had a watch on his wrist and he asked the other Qigong Master if she would place her watch on the table. I had no reason to believe that she was in on a scam, and she had just arrived to town as I had. A Western woman with her got excited and spontaneously took off her watch too, also placing it on the table. The chap sitting at that table was a local Qigong Master known for his unique abilities. He started to breathe heavy and I remember his eyes started to shake and bulge, looking like a Chinese version of Marty Feldman. He really didn't seem like the type who was putting on a show or a scam: he really was deep into whatever he was doing. While he was in what looked like a convulsion, he managed to point to his watch and it appeared that the second-hand had in fact stopped moving. We looked at the other two watches and those second-hands had also had stopped. To my surprise, the wall clock's second-hand was not moving either. As quickly as we noticed all this, the poor guy sitting down slumped in exhaustion and his breathing eventually came back to normal… and the clocks all started moving again. He looked at us and just nodded as if to say, "There, it's done." How do you explain this? If it was a trick, it was a very clever one that to this day I can't explain. We have to simply accept that there are occurrences in this world that simply defy explanation.

Another one of these curiosities was when I led a group of international travelers to the sacred Wu Dang Mountain in China. Up in these mystical mountains is the ancient Taoist Wu Dang Temple renown for being shrouded in mist. I went there with my old friend, the well-respected Qigong Doctor and Master Wan Su Jian, who considered me his "di di" (little brother.) The elder Abbot who headed the temple met us at the gate and thanks to Master Wan's reputation, we were welcomed out of the thick fog into the large room where guests were greeted and offered ceremonial tea. The Abbot told us of his joy to meet us and also his sadness that we couldn't see the spectacular mountains above or the river below as this mist and fog that had been thick for weeks. None of us complained: it was all quite magical just to be there.

I was used to what came next after visiting many temples over the years and lead many, many groups. It was my responsibility to do a ceremonial blessing with the Abbot of the temple for the good luck and health of our group and all the monks who lived at the temple. At Wu Dang, this was quite something as I had to carry lit incense out along a path and then onto an old wooden beam at the edge of a cliff. Imagine walking out to the edge of a swimming pool diving board while blindfolded and you'll get the idea. Of course the mist was so thick that I could barely see my feet and I took small and careful steps. The Abbot walking behind me kept saying , "Zuo la, zuo la" which means "keep going," so I did with absolute trust and many deep Taoist breaths. Now, standing on the edge and feeling like I was floating in open space, I could hear a roaring river below as the Abbot continued his prayers to the local deities. He then said, "Wan lan" signifying the ceremony was done.

When we got back to the group, the Abbot said something to Master Wan that I didn't fully understand, and then he said "Xie, xie" in thanks and walked slowly back to the temple. A person in our group asked Master Wan what the Abbot said before he left. Master Wan, shy but honest, said that the Abbot was happy I didn't fall off the cliff and that it was a good and auspicious sign for us all.

At that moment, Master Wan had an idea and he asked us all to get up and face the river that we could not see but that we could hear. We had less than 10 feet of visibility is that dense, wet fog. We all raised our hands at Master Wan's guidance, and were asked to visualize clarity and light. Facing the Lao Gong points in our palms outward and away toward the sound of the river, we all did the deep breathing we were instructed to do and continued to visualize clarity and light. The exercise seemed like a fun and romantic idea, and I remember some people were getting cold and wanted to go inside.

All of a sudden, the sky opened and rays of warm sunlight poured down on us. It's hard to believe these things as they are occurring, but if any one of the 30 people who was on that trip reads this they will attest to the experience. Only above where we were all standing the mist dissipated and a patch of blue sky appeared. It was quite something. We could now all see where the Abbot made me walk for the ceremony. It was a narrow wooden plank that cantilevered out 15 or 20 feet beyond the edge of a rocky precipice suspended a few hundred feet above the raging river below. No wonder the Abbot said it was auspicious that I hadn't fallen over. The clouds and mist immediately returned. We stayed at the Wu Dang Temple for a couple more days and never again saw even a single ray of sunshine.

I share all of this in what could be a book-full of examples of things that I have seen that are beyond my ability to explain scientifically. I am a very discerning Italian Virgo who is quite skeptical of everything I see. It's my nature to question, and it was this very questioning that allowed me to see Western medicine for what it was and where it was going decades ago that pushed me to look for more effective solutions to healing. It was precisely by deepening my intuitive understanding of the body through my Qigong and Meditation studies that I learned how to heal my own body on many occasions that range from second-degree burns on my hands to multiple bone fractures.

Back in the mid-'70s after studying with a Master healer in Hawaii for a couple of years, I got into a terrible car accident. A head-on collision on the main highway put my head through the windshield and crushed my legs between the hot engine and the body frame. It was a challenge and a gift. It took hours of having the fire department cut my broken body out of the car, after which I was in surgery for six intense hours. I requested no anesthesia so that I could stay alert, observe, and be part of the healing. What I realized was that this "accident" was a perfect opportunity to put the energy healing that I was studying with the Master to use. How many times in life do we face a situation where we are put to the test, to walk our talk and apply what we've been learning. This opportunity was one of them. I took my training in meditative interoception, building an inner sensitivity of what your body is messaging you on the most subtle levels, and used it to support my recovery. I was now laid up in Castle Memorial Hospital in a full body cast, braces and traction. The very first morning after surgery, I woke up and sensed that something was very wrong with my right ankle. My inner vision was that there was an energy block in the joint. Well sure, it was crushed by the car's engine, but it was more than that and I couldn't shake the sense. I soon received a call from the old energy healing teacher I was studying with who was of course shocked to find out what had happened. I told him my sense, and he did some remote viewing and concurred with my conclusion. I asked one of the amazing nurses to let the surgeon know that I wanted to talk with him. When he came into my hospital room, I thanked him and went right into telling him what I was experiencing about the energy block. He said that it was probably true because my talus, metatarsals, and calcaneus were crushed. I said it wasn't that. I told him that I could "see" the broken bones and that there was something more. He actually became livid and tried to leave, but I finally got him to admit that he fused the ankle together with bolts. Although it would never be able to function again, it was "repaired." He went on to say that he was actually renowned in the podiatrist field and was in Honolulu from San Francisco to give a professional lecture on this very technique he performed on me. I told him this approach was unacceptable and I demanded to go back in surgery and have him un-fuse my ankle as I was prepared to heal it myself and have it once again function normally. He actually started yelling and the nurses came in to see this haoli (not-from-the-islands) physician having a fit. He said there already was a chance that I'd never be able to walk again, but if he undid what he had done to my ankle, I absolutely would never be able to stand on it nor walk again in my life. Then he stormed out.

I immediately got on the phone with my teacher who in his 80s was still a licensed psychiatrist. Since psychiatrists are physicians, he got on the phone with the head of the hospital's surgery department he had known for years and arranged for me to go back into surgery. Suffice it to say, the surgeon never said a word to me during the un-fusing surgery and I seem to remember that he hissed when it was done, or un-done in this case.

The following weeks in the hospital, and months in a wheelchair as the body cast was removed in phases, were a dedicated time for me to practice Nei Gong, or "inner work," using visualization. I have many amazing things to share about what took place in that process, but on the day when my teacher casually asked me to stand up out of the wheelchair and get something for him upstairs in his library, I knew it was a challenge. I hadn't stood in months, and I couldn't even exercise because of the casts, so my muscles had atrophied. Yet all the time, and diligently so, I was doing Nei Gong energy healing on myself so I knew that in the deepest sense I was healed... it was just a matter of time for my physical form to catch up. So I looked at my teacher and took the challenge. He had several other students there that day, and they all were in shock. I can remember like it was yesterday when I rolled my wheelchair to the foot of the long staircase in our home that was once Queen Liliuokalani's summer home. I called upon her and all the local spirits, took a deep breath and "saw" my body healthy and strong placing no focus on all the once broken bones in my feet and ankles and knee. I embraced the vision of being immersed in life-force Qi and aligned with the core intention of my body in perfect form and function. I stood up, shaky at first, and grabbed the smooth wooden bannister. I looked up at the long staircase, and started up, one intense step at a time. I remember not stopping, just visualizing the "doing" of it. When I got into the library, I walked past a mirror. It may have been the first time I actually saw myself in months and certainly was the first time standing. There was that body of mine with 40 pounds less weight on it, and weakened by the long recovery. But I was standing. It was a lot to take in all of a sudden and I lost my balance. Right in that moment, which I hadn't realized, my teacher followed me up the stairs and was standing behind me. He held me and slowly guided me to sit in a chair. He said, "Never forget this moment, this sensation of standing and walking. You may not be able to do it again for a while, but you will, it's who you are, who you believe yourself to be."

Anyone who has attended my workshops knows these stories and has seen the many scars on my feet, ankles, and knee. Maybe it was because I questioned these Qi Effect principles of energy healing so deeply in my life that my stubbornness to fully accept them brought me so many opportunities to apply the principles on my own body for self healing. I have also treated many people over the years, from my parents to clients, using these techniques, so I know in my Heart that they are real and that they work. I have also done my share over the years to expose the charlatans that attempt to dupe people into thinking they were everything from gurus to healers. I have little tolerance for those who attempt to manipulate others, especially vulnerable people who are in need of authentic help.

What most of those Qigong Masters at that Beijing convention in the early 1990's were promoting was their ability to send "their Qi" outward from their hands, or minds, to effect change on the world around them. I have a particular opinion about was is referred to as "Qi emission", this idea of collecting "your" Qi and then directing it outward. Some healers may add a caveat here and say it's not "their" Qi they are emitting, but still, they feel that they are emitting Qi none the less.

Qi emission has become an overused and "automatic" statement that was readily adopted by the Western mind and conditioning when Chinese Masters promoted it. Of course the tradition in China uses the term "Wei Qi." Yes, in some circles, this term is focused on the clinical practitioner's "personal" Qi expression and their use of "emitted" Qi, and this in no way the highest level of the term Wei Qi nor its application. From my personal experience, it does not serve the practitioner who focuses on this. I've seen many Qigong "Masters" in China (and outside of China) who focus on this approach actually die at an early age. Yes, I have personally met these people (all men by the way). They all boasted about their ability to "collect" Qi, build it in sufficient concentration, and then emit it through the the point in their palms known as Lao Gong points. When I found out that many of these Qigong Masters died in their 50s and 60s, it really made me wonder. I have also noticed curious energetic/emotional anomalies in non-Chinese clinical practitioners around the world who focus on Qi emission. This word comes from the Latin "emittere" which as you can guess, means "to send out" like the exhaust pipe of a car. It's not the best association when it comes to healing.

I feel that for an empowered Qigong clinical practitioner to place their focus on the fact that they are sending out "their" Qi, or any Qi, is not empowering for them or their patients. It may sound good and exotic, and "sick" people are happy to "receive" whatever they can receive, but, in the long run, it's not empowering for them either.

How can you "emit" Qi when we are immersed in an infinite field of this life force energy? We made the case that Qi doesn't even exist in this dimension we exist in, and we can't realistically subject it to the physics of space/time by saying it can "move" from one place to another. Even if you try to argue that Qi is in this dimension (which of course no one can prove), if it is in infinite supply and presence, how in the world can you move infinity? If people could only understand the depths of the Qi Effect principle of activating the Qi/"physical" relationship at the quantum level, things would be very different in a positive way. Healers, by changing their language away from "emitting," would step out of their dualistic and ego-bias and embrace that they were in fact activating the Qi Effect. Patients, and everyone for that matter, would come to understand that they too are immersed in an infinite potentiality field of this life force energy and that they have full access to activating Qi themselves. This is a much more empowering and egalitarian view that I believe is much more in line with what the ancients sensed to be true.

I visited both Shi Yuan Hospital and the Shanghai Qigong Hospital in China and spent time in both facilities at length. I mention these because they were relatively large government-influenced institutions and both focused on a "medicine-less" approach to healing with an emphasis on Qi emission protocols used by their resident doctors. Though they both had relatively good success at helping people according to what they told me, I noticed two things. First, their patients came to them to get healed in the very same, disempowering way of any Western medical facility. There was not much sense of supporting the patient by reviewing their lifestyle issues or emotional challenges. Symptoms and life situations were discussed briefly, and then patients would sit in chairs along with sometimes dozens of other patients and a Qigong doctor would go around "emitting Qi" to heal them.

There were individual doctors who would, in confidence, tell me that they weren't using their "personal Qi" but were connecting with a more Universal Qi… and yes, these were typically the doctors that spent more time talking with the patients to learn more about them. I realize that there are Medical Qigong practitioners all around the world today that have attempted to learn Qi emission techniques and also embrace a good and caring attitude. The challenge is that there is still an inherent belief that Qi is being emitted in some way or another, and this creates a situation where there is a "sender" and a "receiver." Implicit in this arrangement is the sense that the "sender" is losing some Qi, at some level, and that they will need to replenish their supply. Also implicit is that the "receiver" doesn't have enough Qi or that the quality of their Qi is weak, out of balance or drained. Even if the supposed Qi-emitting healer feels as if they are emitting universal Qi, they still claim that they are the "emitters" and as such, they are claiming access to Qi and its manipulation. You may call this just semantics, but I believe it is fundamental.

I pointed out those two institutions because they were established, long-running operations. Many, many individual Medical Qigong practitioners operating out of small clinics around the world adhere to these same principles. I've met many of these practitioners who carry the "Container" world view and were constantly working to replenish their Qi reserves or their ability to access Qi. I've also met many otherwise healthy doctors younger than 60 years old who fall ill or have emotional issues.

These practitioners are generally good people with generally good intentions, but I feel that they have deep misperceptions as to what is really taking place. There are other experienced Chinese Medicine doctors who agree with me. It's natural for most people to stick with "accepted" perceptions that have become comfortable, especially when many of these concepts in Qigong have roots that go back in Taoist and Buddhist history hundreds if not thousands of years. It is also a romantic notion to believe that the ancients had all the answers. Some will even trace these concepts of "building," "storing" and "emitting" Qi back to the fabled Yellow Emperor of China many thousands of years ago. These are great stories, but they also came from a time when science and culture was very different than today. To me, it's not the role of a leader in any field to simply follow tradition. It is our responsibility to constantly question and revisit even the most comfortable notions, especially those that can't be scientifically proven like Qi emission.

I did study with two Qigong Masters in China who I greatly respect and who used "emitted" Qi in their healing treatments. One was a devout Taoist, a respected Traditional Chinese Medicine (TCM), and Classical Chinese Medicine (CCM) doctor who treated some of the top CCP government officials and business leaders in China. During the two years that I lived and studied in his clinic, I saw these types of people come to the clinic and was always asked to stay in my room with the curtains drawn so I wasn't seen. Being the first and only Westerner to live at that clinic, it would not have been looked upon as a good thing to have me there to witness who came for treatments.

What made this Master unique was that he was very clear with me that it wasn't "his personal" Qi that he was emitting. It was because of this critical factor that I studied with him those years, and continued for another 25 years. His intention, when he directed his "transmitting" Lao Gong point in his palm to a patient, was to keep his other Lao Gong point in his other hand facing upward. This was to allow himself to be a conduit for Qi flow. I participated in daily healing sessions with him and his Qi healer trainees and worked on hundreds of clients over the years and experienced many positive results. To me, this felt a lot closer to what was really taking place energetically, but it still didn't sit with me as the complete explanation of what was taking place.

I still do not completely agree with this technique of "emitted Qi," and have many examples to explain why I feel it is neither safe nor healthy to embrace. Yes, the intention is beautiful and it is very seductive, but without a critical shift to fully understand what I am sharing in the Qi Effect principles, neither the practitioner nor the recipient patient will benefit in the long run.

From what I have studied, experienced, intuited, and trust, "Wei Qi" is the electromagnetic energy field that is entangled (from a Quantum Physics perspective) between the Clinical Practitioner and the "patient" and the space/time field effect all around us individually as well. Wei Qi is not directly Qi, since as I have shared in the Qi Effect principles, Qi does not exist in this dimension. Please let someone measure it or show me that I'm wrong and I will gladly concede. They can't.

This electromagnetic field around us is real and is in this dimension. It can be measured both with classical Newtonian physics measurements and substantiated to the 'nth degree in all quantum physics measurements and experiments. Every atom carries an electromagnetic field, so of course, every person, animal, gaseous cloud, liquid, and solid object carries with it an electromagnetic Wei Qi field. This is not to be construed as Qi.

Here's the good part though… This Wei Qi field is quantum entangled with Qi inter-dimensionally. I know this starts to sound eccentric, but go back to the Qi Effect chapter to review all the science that I have shared. This is critically important to the Qi Effect principles. If you wish to cling to the accepted notion that you are a "Qi collector" and that you emit Qi, that's fine. The reason I feel we need to shift out of that notion is that it is very limiting and disempowering. Not only have I personally witnessed Qigong Masters dying from practicing this, but I have seen others display unhealthy expressions of what happens when you harbor a belief system that you build a storehouse of life-force energy and then selectively send it out to others (or rice paddies) and then have to work to collect more, and repeat the process over and over again. What we carry in our world view defines the world we view.

Using Wei Qi to "facilitate" healing does not mean the practitioner is "sending out" their Qi or even universal Qi. Of course this can "appear" to be so and from a certain limited perspective, this looks like what is taking place. But that's like saying "I cheered for my team and they won the game." I'm oversimplifying, but I hope you get what I mean. I am very sensitive to healers falling prey to ego and duality. It's seductive and convenient to take only a sliver of the truth and use it to your advantage. It's better to seek a deeper explanation of why energy healers actually facilitate and inspire healing in others. This is a beautiful offering that helps many and I feel it can help many more, including the healers, if they can embrace the depths of what I am sharing here.

How we explore this sacred cow of emitted Qi is up to you, and I feel it's my responsibility to bring it up as part of our exploration of the Qi Effect curiosities.

What I suggest is that you simply allow the possibility that what "appears" to be Qi emission to be the activation of the Qi Effect. This means that the healer/clinician is facilitating the quantum entanglement (and the concept of quantum tunneling). As the "observer" influencing the field effect and wave function, the naturally occurring Qi Effect is activated at a higher amplitude and more effective level. It is consciousness and awareness that collapses the wave function. This is the amazing influence of the "observer effect." In Quantum physics, the wave function describes every situation, and yes, most times these situations take place at the atomic or subatomic level. Since we are all made of atoms, the wave function still describes the relationship between healer and patient at some level. The wave function describes the field of possibilities. In other words, this is the many possible outcomes of any interaction. This field of possible outcomes "collapses" and becomes the outcome based on the view, intention, and belief system of the observer. Can you see the importance of what beliefs the healer carries and how that influences the outcome of the healing process?

Shifting our relationship with Qi in this way is much more Heart-centered, nd much less egotistical and dualistic. It is also the final, and what I feel, critical step in disengaging the powerful and effective energy healing arts from the Intellectual Mind and patriarchal dominance of conditioned thinking. We can easily be duped into thinking that since we are dealing with something as exotic and alternative as Qi energy healing that we would be outside of the conditioning set into our epigenetic programming for five centuries. True and lasting healing (and personal practice involving the same energy principle set) can only take place when we disengage from duality. This means both the healer/patient duality as well as the "my Qi/your Qi" duality. It seems subtle, but it is critical for our evolution.

The fact is, whether we are speaking of clinical Qi healing or the personal practice of Qigong, Reiki, or any other types of energy healing, the research supporting the positive healing effects are impossible to question. As Chairman of the non-profit Qigong Institute, I am proud of the work our President Tom Rogers does as a volunteer to collect research studies being done around the world for our free "Qigong & Energy Medicine Database™." If you are interested in doing your own exploration, visit www.QigongInstitute.org and type in any word relating to health. You will find data to show how the Qi Effect expresses itself to hardcore medical researchers from top universities. It's undeniable that the practices that make Qigong what it is (conscious breathing, gentle movement and stretching, and calm, mental focus) are able to reduce stress, bring the body-mind-spirit into alignment. Qigong helps bring a person back to homeostasis: the natural, healthy state of being.

It is important to remember the debilitating effect that stress has on our body, mind, and spirit. Stress can range from cellular stress to emotional stress, and wherever it is expressed, danger lurks. As the National Institutes of Health (NIH) in the U.S. states, over 70% of all disease and illness is stress-related. Whatever Qigong does to reduce and manage stress has a direct and positive effect on our health and well-being.

Telomeres are the bits of protein and DNA at the end of your chromosomes that help protect your DNA each time it replicates so that the process is done correctly and there are no genetic mutations leading to things like cancer or cell death. Of course, each time any of your cells replicate in a process call mitosis, the DNA must replicate as well (meiosis.) Telomeres have been found to get shorter as we age, and it is accepted scientific fact that their length is a reliable biomarker for aging. Curiously, research shows that practices like Qigong, Tai Chi, Yoga, and Meditation help maintain telomere length, and theses practices do this through their ability to both reduce stress and inflammation and help us manage our homeostasis. I have to add that in a 2016 study with 4,780 nurses it was found that those who regularly drank coffee had verifiably longer telomeres! This is not to dissuade you from doing Qigong or other empowering practices, but just imagine if you did and you drank coffee… It is common sense that less stress leads to a healthier body, mind, and spirit, and this keeps us feeling young and vital. Dr. Ken Sancier, founder of the Qigong Institute, wrote a seminal paper in 1996 on the anti-aging benefits of Qigong and I urge you to check it out. Not only is the reduction of oxidative stress on a cellular level at work here by these simple practices, but the increased ability to activate the Qi Effect.

Cancer killed more people in the U.S. than confirmed SARS-Cov2 deaths in 2020. 606,520 cancer deaths, with 1,806,590 new cancer cases diagnosed in that year according to the government website PubMed. Curiously, any treatment for the over 100 different types of cancer that is not approved by various government agencies makes them illegal and thus prohibits physicians from recommending them or using them in treatment. To me, this is a very sad state of affairs as we know so many natural and non-invasive solutions exist around the world that are shown to be effective.

Qigong is not a "treatment" for cancer, but study after study shows its ability through intentional breathing techniques to oxygenate blood. This helps in oxidizing anaerobic cancer cells and has an inhibitory effect on cancer growth, both in vitro and in vivo studies. Add to this Qigong's ability to lower and manage stress and bring the body to a natural state of homeostasis, and it is clear that Qigong is key to supporting those facing cancer, especially while they are undergoing challenging treatments so hard on the human body like chemotherapy and radiation. Giving people the understanding that they can and do contribute to their healing process is one of the great benefits of Qigong. Of course, when our body is in an extreme chaotic state such as it is during a disease trauma, we actually have a boosted ability to activate the Qi Effect. It only makes sense then to move out of the victimization mentality that so often debilitates those facing disease and remember this heightened ability to heal. I remind those challenged by cancer or any dis-ease that even though it may not seem so, you have a great opportunity to activate Qi in your body and energy field during your illness. Those who can tap into this are the ones that surprise physicians with "spontaneous healing" as I have seen many, many times with clients. I've even seen it with my own father when he was facing bladder cancer and totally eliminated any cancer markers in his blood after only three weeks of practice, causing his oncologist to have to cancel surgery at the hospital when he did the pre-op blood test! Curiously, my Dad doesn't even believe in Qigong! But, as Nobel Laureate Niels Bohr said about his "lucky" horse shoe over the door of his office, "Of course I don't believe it—but I've sometimes noticed that it works even when you don't believe in it!"

The vagus nerve, a critical part of our central nervous system located in our lower abdominal area, is receiving more and more attention by the medical community in recent years. When activated, it seems to harmonize nerve impulse flow with the sinoatrial nerve in the heart to increase Heart Rate Variability (HRV). Increased HRV is proven to boost our ability to deal with stressful situations and through Qigong's deep, abdominal breathing techniques, the vagus nerve is activated in such a way that it positively triggers the sinoatrial nerve in the heart.

As I continue to point out, these bio-physiological observations, whether they relate to neural activity, biochemical action, or cell function, are simply what we can see with our current scientific technologies through the lens of our belief system and conditioning. I know that as technology and beliefs advance, we will come to find that the Qi Effect is in fact activated during healing, and it's potential actually rises during illness. Of course, as I've pointed out, we can't yet measure Qi, but for those of us around the world who understand this with our Intuitive Mind insights, we are benefiting greatly by our practices that help us align, ground, and center our electromagnetic Wei Qi energy field. This is what increases the Qi Effect by activating Qi and this life-force relationship to our body/energy field.

The ancients guided us but they didn't define us or dictate how we should practice. They brilliantly took us to the limits of where they were in their times, and it is for us to continue that intention, and take our practice and insights to the amazing limits where we are now in our times. This is a journey of exploration and discovery that will continue to the end of time.

I feel that it is critical that we recognize this concept of "activating Qi" and how that activation not only brings the physical health of our being to vibrancy, but how the energetic aspects of our being becomes a more conscious expression of our every day. This shift from the belief that we "move" or "affect" Qi towards the understanding that we are actually activating the relationship between Qi and our physical/energetic body changes so much about how we practice Qigong or any energy healing practice.

When we begin sensing the Yin and Yang qualities of various Qigong movements and positions, it is a start at understanding both the phases and spacial dynamics of where we are placing our hands, arms, legs, head, etc. These various positions create energetic dynamics that activate Qi in different ways and why certain moves are more effective than others and why some strengthen and heal specific Organ Systems the way they do. What many Qigong, Tai Qi, Yoga, and other instructors don't fully understand is the 4-dimensional geometry created by where the Lao Gong (in your palms), Yong Chuan (bottom of your feet), Dan Tians (head, chest, belly), Bai Hui (top of your head), etc. are in their interrelationship in Cartesian space... This may sound advanced or complex, but it really isn't. Essentially I am reminding us that the placement of our body when we are practicing these exercises creates an energetic effect in the three-dimensional space of our physical body AND the forth-dimension that we can say is the energetic body, what the Taoist refer to as the Wei Qi Field. Just as the position/distance of your smart phone to a router affects the number of WiFi bars that show up - or the position of a magnet affects the array of iron filings around it - the position and orientation of our body - and all those key acupoints/energy spots distributed throughout our body - deeply affects how we engage with our Wei Qi Field and thus, how we activate Qi.

This is not seen nor recognized by many who play/practice Qigong, yet it can be experienced in Wuji Hundun Qigong from Master Duan Zhi Liang as well as the Organ Cleansing Qigong (Zang Fu Gong) style, both of which I choose to focus on when I teach precisely because of this fact. This is why I remind people that the Wuji Hundun form is "shamanic" in nature; it is not just a bunch of random movements. Most don't fully understand this but it's helpful we at least hear this as it opens our Intuitive Mind. The shamanic quality essentially means that you dynamically position your physical body in the Wei Qi field - and this in relationship with the nature and environment around you including trees, water, mountains, Cardinal Points, etc. - and listen how your orientation actually aligns the whole of the field itself. This is in part how the energy signatures of the Organ Systems that extend into the field are brought into coherence and integration. This perspective of alignment and clearing is much more effective and useful to humans than being trapped in the Five Element Model of "energy management" that is so easily grabbed on by neo-Taoists.

To fully embrace this we are asked to keep playing and listening as we do our practice. Watching and seeing your movements in this 4D space (3D Cartesian + energetic) by becoming more and more sensitive to your Intuitive Mind and not overthinking with your Intellectual Mind is key.

The Wei Qi field is essentially what we would call a hologram. A hologram is defined as an "image that contains information which can produce the whole of a 3D space." The word hologram was coined by the 1971 Nobel Prize in Physics winner Denis Gabor, so remember that this concept is steeped in pretty basic science and not as "out there" as you may think. Hologram comes from the Greek "holos" or "whole" and "gram" which essentially means "to write." So we can think of a hologram as a space that can define (write) the whole of the space itself from any point in that space. I can remember visiting the famous Museum of Holography in New York City back in the 1970s and being fascinated by the holograms. You could peer into the corner of one of these projected or glass holograms and from that corner, look into the farthest edge of the whole image. What was even more fascinating was a display where one glass hologram was broken and a corner piece was cracked off. You could pick it up and look into this dislocated piece of the hologram and it still contained the whole image if you held if up to your eye.

The Wei Qi Field is very much like this. Any point in the space around us immersed in our personal Wei Qi Field contains the whole of the energy field itself. Although our various Organ Systems from the Heart to the Liver projects its unique and specific energetic signature into the whole of the Wei Qi Field, any point in the field reflects in some way, the totality of all the Organ Systems. This unified, holographic field perspective of our personal energy field will help you in many ways. For one, wherever you move your physical body during your practice, it will influence the whole of the holographic field. This means that you don't have to overly concern yourself with the specifics of "where" these Organ energy signatures reside, and focus more on the power of your intention to positively affect them for healing, strengthening, and rejuvenation. Secondly, embracing the holographic truth of the Wei Qi Field will help you build your sensitivity as to why you position your hands, arms, legs, torso, head, etc. in the specific postures of a Qigong move. Learning to breathe into this sensitivity will help you improve your ability to activate Qi since certain postures and refined positioning of your Lao Gong points in relationship to your Dan Tians, Jing Mai (acupuncture meridians), and the Wei Qi Field itself do this better than others.

Trust this and keep feeling into all this with the awareness that your Wei Qi Field has a dynamic toroidal structure. The torus is a donut-shaped, 3D structure. It is not fixed and rigid, but dynamically moving from it's chaotically neutral core where Yin and Yang dance to it's outward "donut" edges where Yin and Yang are at their extremes. Discovering that our Heart resonant "core" resides in the center of the torus teaches us that making peace with chaos is essential on this journey of being human. This is where Qigong is meant to take us... beyond simply a physical experience but truly one that positively influences our mind and spirit as well.

Our toroidal Wei Qi Field is a microcosm of the Earth's Wei Qi field... The Earth's Wei Qi Field is a microcosm of the solar system's Wei Qi Field... the solar system's Wei Qi Field is a microcosm of the Milky Way galactic Wei Qi Field, which of course is a microcosm of the Universe itself. This fractal nature of embedded and interwoven fields is the nature of our existence... and when we embrace this in a conscious way, we increase our probability of activating Qi. This is the essence of the Qi Effect. As we come into the awareness of our sovereign, infinitely-reflected nature of all that is around and through us, we start to discover the truth of who we are and what it means to find our purpose as humans - and how we can better relate to others around us with Heart resonance and kindness. When we breathe into this, meditate on this, weave this into our personal practice, our alignment is empowering and our resources for healing, rejuvenation, and transformation become more and more accessible..

Qi Effect Exercises

The Qi Effect is more than a theory, it really is a basic principle of life on planet Earth. Like any principle, it should be put to the scientific test so to speak. This means that each one of us should put it into a real-world application if we truly wish to benefit.

The following exercises are intended to assist you in putting these Qi Effect concepts to work in your daily experience. Have fun exploring these and observe how you feel. Observe what you see inside you, observe what seems to shift around you. Remember that every shift we make in our world view shifts the world we view. If you have questions on any of these exercises, check out our online videos and Courses at the non-profit www.CommunityAwake.com website with its many online offerings. If you feel so inspired, attend one of our workshops to go more in-depth into the subtleties of these empowering exercises.

1) The Qi Effect Mantra

First and foremost, I feel it is important to set intention and focus in our life. Without aligning our energy and Intuitive Mind Heart Resonance focus toward an intention, we will be like a bottle floating in the turbulent sea of the Survival and Intellectual Mind. As a fun exercise, you may want to learn what I'll call the Qi Effect "mantra." This is the core intention-setting principles that describe the Qi Effect itself. Though the ancient Sanskrit word "mantra" is typically associated with a sacred utterance, the fact is that the etymological root of mantra is "man-" which simply means "to think." In the Middle Vedic period in India (1,000 BCE - 500 BCE), mantras became a true blend of art, science, and spirituality. It is in that spirit of realizing the power of intention that I offer this mantra to help you align the power of your mind and focus to think in an empowering way.

Qi Effect Mantra

"I embrace my immersion in the infinite field of Qi and I activate the Qi Effect at my cellular, molecular, and atomic levels, to sustain my healed self, for my rejuvenation, insights, and transformation."

I suggest you find a quiet place where you are by yourself and with minimal disturbance for 20 minutes or so. Turn off your phone and music. Write this mantra down on a piece of paper in your own handwriting and hold it while you gaze at the words. Read this mantra four or five times, and then close your eyes. Try repeating it from memory. Observe where you missed any of it, and read it again until you can repeat it effortlessly from memory with closed eyes.

As you repeat this mantra, allow it to find a natural place in your Intuitive mind. You may observe that it becomes a discrete set of concepts such as Who, What, Where, Why, and When. Allow your wonderful Intellectual Mind to do its thing if this is the case… then return to your breath, and Heart Resonance.

As you repeat this mantra, you may find yourself asking why you are doing it, or questioning how that saying words will even help. Allow your hard working Survival Mind to engage however it feels, but keep coming back to your Heart-centered Intuitive Mind.

As you continue to repeat this mantra, you may have a glimpse or sensation that you have heard it before. Maybe it is that you have known this mantra, or parts of it, for a long time. You have a sense of familiarity. This is when our Intuitive Mind is finally engaged. Stay with this sensation.

This is where you will find your groove and attain the deepest benefits. When our Intellectual Mind and our Survival Mind finally stabilize (usually they do this when they feel safe and listened to) they will back down from your mental engagement and your Intuitive Mind will become the primary mental bandwidth involved in your mantra repetition. This is key.

When our Intuitive Mind becomes the primary thinking process, you basically have hijacked the sabotaging effect of the Survival and Intellectual Minds. When they no longer play out their programming, you will start to discover a level of freedom to explore two key areas where only the Intuitive Mind can take you.

First, it takes your Mind into the Akasha. I use this Sanskrit word since we are already using the word mantra. The Akasha refers to "open space" or simply, "to be." When Intuitive Mind opens to the Akasha, we receive insights, information, and awareness that may not seem normal. The Ancient Greeks used the term "metanoia" for a "transformed mind" that would occur at times of insight. This is why we must activate and immerse ourselves in our Intuitive Mind from time to time as it will open us to our potential and help us see our lives, our health, and our challenges in new ways.

As Einstein is attributed to having said, "We cannot solve our problems with the same thinking we used when we created them." I like that quote, but there is no proof that Eistein ever said it. Most likely it was Ram Dass who said it back in 1970. Discover what emerges from within you when you tap into the Akasha. Keep repeating this mantra and see where it takes you.

Another technique can be to read this quote over and over slowly and record yourself doing that. You can also listen to one of my several Guided Meditations on this that I have online. Of course there is a difference between repeating a mantra to yourself and listening to a recorded mantra. The fact is, there is a tradition for both techniques. Some people can simply drop into their Intuitive Mind easier if they listen and don't speak or even subvocalize. Experiment either way and see what brings you the best results and the most joy.

The second place immersing into your Intuitive Mind can take you is your subconscious. Just as your Survival and Intellectual Mind can sabotage you with their structured and programmed ways, your subconscious is the master of this disturbance. It's been programmed your whole life: most of the time without you even knowing it. It has also been programmed epigenetically before your life, thanks to the conscious and subconscious influences of your parents and ancestors. Some of these "programs" are helpful, but most of them are typically associated with the extremes of trauma and survival-related experiences. That is why they have endured for the generations. What is most destructive is that they influence you without your clear knowledge or awareness. Since you typically can't do much about them, they control you.

When you activate the Qi Effect and wake up your Intuitive Mind, you increase your ability to gain access to your subconscious. When you have access to these otherwise intangible influences on your life, you have half a chance of changing them into more positive influences, or stopping them all together.

Repeat the Qi Effect Mantra, or listen to a recording of it, until you find yourself in the open space of your Intuitive Mind. From that point, the adventure will be up to you.

2) Spiral Breathing

Breathing techniques have long been part of practices that remove us from the trappings of "ordinary" mental activity. Whether these be Shamanic breathing practices or spiritual breathing techniques from Hinduism, Buddhism, Islamic, Taoism, or esoteric Judeo-Christian origins, using the breath is a very tangible way to activate the Qi Effect.

Spiral Breathing is a technique that I have developed which brings together many principles that I've learned from studies around the world with Masters in many different cultures. It is not tied to any religion or system; it simply uses solid, scientific and common-sense principles that have affected positive results in the many people I've shared it with in workshops I offer.

The use of circular and spiral movement has origins that go back to the beginnings of recorded history on this planet. Whether it be from the Druid tradition or temple dances in Sumeria over 5,000 years ago, movement in a circular way is a natural mirroring of what we see in the orbiting heavenly bodies like the Moon and planets. It is natural that the ancient wisdom holders would honor the circle through the Ancient Greeks with Pythagoras and on to the amazing Islamic mathematicians of the Middle Ages. With the tools of modern technology, we can peer into the Universe and see how spiral and elliptical movement is a basic function of celestial trajectories. We can also look deep into our cellular structure and observe the DNA helix, atomic structure and spherical electron clouds.

When we use circles, spirals, and the torus in this Spiral Breathing exercise, we are tapping into a basic principal of the world around us. We will be supported by it by being in alignment with it.

First, get into a comfortable sitting position. Yes, you can do this lying down or standing, but if you can I suggest you start with sitting. No, you don't need to get into a full lotus sitting posture with your legs crossed, but if you are able and it makes you happy, go for it. I like to sit in a half-lotus position myself as it keeps my back straight and helps me align my lower abdominal core. If you'd rather sit in a chair, try not to lean against the chair back as this will weaken your core muscles. Choose a more alert and present-minded posture by sliding your butt a little more to the front edge of the chair and sit in a relaxed, but upright position.

With your shoulders relaxed, legs uncrossed and feet flat on the ground, allow your hands to rest relaxed on your thighs. You can hold your fingers in a mudra if you like. Do whatever makes you feel comfortable.

Start by taking a deep inhale breath (pushing out your belly if you can and extending your abdomen outward) and only then slightly raise your chest as you continue your inhale. When you've completed as full of an inhale as you are able, exhale deeply by allowing your chest to drop and gently squeeze your abdominal muscles to help push your diaphragm up against your lungs to push out what's left of your breath. Try this a few times to get used to this empowering diaphragmatic breathing.

Place the tip of your tongue against your hard pallet. This is that area just above your upper row of teeth. Keep the pressure gentle but connected throughout this whole exercise. This will help engage your Heart.

Take your next deep inhale and guide your focus to the area sometimes called your Third Eye. Imagine this spot between your eyebrows and a little inside your head. This is the area of the powerful Pineal Gland and the core energetic and neurological functions of your brain. It is also the realm of the Crown Chakra in Yogic studies and the Upper Dan Tian in Qigong practice. Whatever your knowledge base or your personal practice is, fine: enjoy your Mind. For this practice we simply use this spot as one of our core anchor points for our spiral.

When your inhale is complete and fully resident at your Third Eye, begin your exhale very slowly. As you exhale, imagine it is traveling downward and around your body in a spiral trajectory all the way to your tailbone. It really doesn't matter whether this is in a clockwise or counter-clockwise direction although some will have a fit by me saying this. These directions are all relative and depend on your point of view. If you really need to hold onto this belief about direction, then pick a direction as you wish.

Depending on the length of your breath and your ability to visualize the "distance" from the top of your head to your tailbone in a spiraling motion path around your body, you may find the need to do this exercise with two sequences of inhales and exhales. This is ok, but you may find it more effective to practice a bit until you can "travel" from your Third Eye to your tailbone in a single, deep exhale, even if you have to speed up the spiral motion. Practice this until you are comfortable, each time guiding your inhale back to your Third Eye.

As you use your visualization and guide your breath from your head down and around your body, tap into your imagination and be creative. Try and "see" the various parts of your body as you travel that downward spiral. There is an ancient Taoist saying in the Qigong writings that in Mandarin Chinese goes like this: "Yi Tao, Qi Tao." It translates literally to, "Mind Way, Qi Way." Some have translated this to "Where the Mind goes, the Qi goes." I rather translate this (after having studied this phrase for some 30 years) as, "The Way of the Mind, is the Way of Qi." This has brought me to a new and much more empowering way of understanding this. "Yi" literally means "bring Qi to Mind" as we do with a memory or an intention. "Tao" can mean a "path, a way" or a natural journey. Understanding this simple but incredibly powerful concept can support your Spiral Breathing practice immensely.

As you visualize your various body parts during your spiral trajectory, imagine that simply by bringing your Yi attention and focus to your shoulder, your Liver, or your spine, you are "activating" the Qi Effect at that spot. This is what this whole book is about. Tapping into the power of your Mind, your "Yi," to activate the relationship between Qi and your physical body is what will wake up the healing ability that you were born with. It simply has been latent, if not dormant, because of the limited thinking and destructive programming of a world that has been run from the Survival and Intellectual Mind for millennia.

Continue this first part of the Spiral Breathing exercise for a while until it comes naturally. Wherever your Intuitive Mind "lands" on your different body parts is fine. If it is different each journey of the downward spiral, fine. If you keep landing on the same body part, organ, area, that is fine too. This is your journey. Embrace it, allow it. Use the basic principles that I offer here, but make it your own. Allowing yourself that freedom will not only make it more fun and flexible, but it will invite you to continue and explore where this exercise can ultimately take you.

The second part of this exercise is about bringing in some specific energy points throughout your body that you may like to work with during the downward spiral exhale. Again, this is your journey to discover what works best for you, but I will share with you some powerful and effective approaches to this exercise that work for me and others.

When you begin your exhale and travel the downward spiral, try including both Lungs - going "through" one and then the other along the spiral trajectory. Do the same with the Kidneys - going through one and then the other. Then go through your reproductive organs - going through your gonads, one side then the other. Terminate your spiral at your Perineum while squeezing your anal sphincter at the end of your exhale.

Repeat this breathing and visualization sequence until it becomes natural… and then we can go on to the next step.

When you are comfortable with guiding your exhale breath to your Perineum while squeezing your anal sphincter, visualize your focus moving a bit upwards to your Lower Dantian (located a couple of inches below your navel, and a little bit internal to your belly.) The exercise here is to hold the squeeze while your are at the very end of your exhale while simultaneously bringing your attention to the Lower Dantian. Practice this until you feel comfortable, and then we'll go to the final phase of the exhale portion of this exercise.

When you feel you have successfully brought your breath focus to your Lower Dantian, then we can move on. Remember that this is not an exact spot but is a high-probability energetic location. You are asked to feel into this region and trust.

Once you can guide your exhale from your Third Eye down the spiral through your Lungs, Kidneys, gonads and then up to your Lower Dantian, the final step is to move your Yi focus directly back to your spine, to a point known as the Ming Men point. Doing this exercise effectively will complete your full exhale starting at your Third Eye and ending at your Ming Men.

The Ming Men is known in Acupuncture as DU-4 (Du Meridian 4 or also Governing Vessel 4) and is translated from Mandarin as "Life Gate." If the ancient Taoists gave this point that name, you know it has great power. The Ming Men is located below the spinous process of Lumbar Vertebra 2 and it is a powerful point for tonifying the Kidney System by activating Jing Qi, and benefiting the spine and legs. Read more about this if you wish to learn Acupuncture specifics. What you are doing in the Spiral Breathing exercise will create Qi activation in a similar way, and for some people, it can be just as effective as having a needle treatment. Explore.

You have completed your full exhale pathway for the Spiral Breathing exercise. Now we must return your breath to the starting point, your Third Eye, to complete the cycle.

Once your Yi focus has followed your exhale down your spiral to your Ming Men point and you are completely empty of breath, begin your inhale by directing your focus to your Vagus Nerve, located in the center of your lower abdomen within your gut. From the Vagus Nerve, create an energetic pathway to your heart (there is actually a physical nerve pathway along the sinoatrial nerve directly inside your heart.) Continuing your inhale, allow your focus to travel to where the tip of your tongue has been gently touching your hard palette. Finally, your inhale returns home to your Third Eye, in the energetic region of your Upper Dantian and physical locale of your Pineal Gland.

Try practicing just your inhale phase, repeating it over and over until you can "feel" and "see" through interoception your Yi visualization traveling this inner pathway from your Ming Men, through your Vagus nerve, inside your heart, through your tongue tip, and deep into your Third Eye.

Now, let's tie your exhale and inhale together to create one full breath cycle. Your exhale follows your downward spiral, and your inhale energetically links the grounding of your Ming Men/Lower Dantian through your Heart Center/Middle Dantian and back to your Third Eye/ Upper Dantian. Keep experimenting with this. The more you put into this, the more you will discover. Once you are comfortable with what I've outlined here, feel free to "customize" this exercise and include other organs or body parts into your exhaling downward spiral.

These exercises are meant to be practical and put to the test. If you are facing some health challenge, include that organ, body region, or function in your spiral trajectory. I know people who use this for emotional challenges as well. Energy is energy. Allow your spiral to move through any emotion that you are facing and then include that emotion in your inhale to transform it in your Heart Resonance field. Surprise yourself at what you are capable of achieving. Trust.

Visit www.CommunityAwake.com if you would like to take the online Course on Spiral Breathing and learn through audio and video support material, which includes how to gently move your body and also goes into the advanced toroidal Wei Qi energy field around our body and how to access it.

For some, this type of Nei Gong or "inner exercise" visualization is easy. For others, it can be a challenge. Be gentle wherever you are with this, and keep playing with it (rather than "working" on it) until you feel as if you are watching yourself in a movie or experiencing a pleasant sensation. There is more and more scientific research proving the power of visualization. Whether it is what you hear about how Olympic athletes visualize shaving 100ths of a second off their times, or it is what you hear about people healing their ailments through mental exercises, we know that biological/medical science is starting to understand the power of our mind to affect positive change on our body, emotions, and spirit.

3) Organ Cleansing Qigong - Zang Fu Gong - Qi Activation

Organ Cleansing Qigong (also known by the Mandarin Chinese name "Zang Fu Gong") is a powerful style of Qigong practiced by many thousands of people around the world that will dramatically shift your perspective on how your view your body and your various organ systems. 18 specific Qigong moves address physical, emotional, and energetic aspects of each of your organ systems, teaching you how to transform your physical health and your emotion response tendencies to bring your body, mind, and spirit into optimal alignment, grounding, and healing.

I created this Qigong form after living in China and studying many different forms from various elder Masters. Thousands of people attest to its effectiveness and I am honored by the 200 Qigong Instructors that I have personally certified to teach it around the world.

This Qigong form incorporates specific breathing, gentle movement and stretching, and positive, intentional imaging to help heal and strengthen our body, mind, and spirit. It is best to watch it on video or take a class. My YouTube Channel has a couple of videos on this https://www.youtube.com/c/FrancescoGarripoli, and www.CommunityAwake.com has info on my workshops and online Courses.

4) Mind Alignment

It is natural for random thoughts to intrude into our practice... Qigong is of course a form of moving meditation, so many times a practice session serves as my "meditation time" as well. When random thoughts enter, I first allocate them to either my Survival Mind or my Intellectual Mind, then I typically say "thank you"... and let that aspect of my Mind know it has no place in my Qigong or meditation practice. I may also ask if the thought is "useful in this moment" or if I need to "take action on it in this moment." Typically, the answer is "No" and that is a way to gently place it aside for later processing. I will always say "Thank you" again so that I can invite my Heart to stay engaged and keep my Intuitive Mind activated. This is a simple, but very powerful exercise as a "first aid" for mental intrusion. Emotion Alchemy is the practice for actually processing the emotions that come up for full transformation: I teach workshops on this technique I developed. This Mind Alignment exercise is very helpful to maintain calm centering. Enjoy!

Visit www.CommunityAwake.com to explore the Guided Meditations there and learn through audio and video support material in the online Courses.

5) Heart Resonance

Look at the world around you and ask yourself at what level your Heart is fully engaged.

In a world that has seemingly gone mad with all the divisiveness we've been seeing in the past years, reminders to stay Heart-centered are more important than ever. Curiously, "divisiveness" can only exist in the world when it exists inside us first. It's easy to "blame" the world, blame leaders, blame politics... but the truth is, transforming our inner battles into a more Heart-aligned way of being is key.

Probably the most meaningful way to bring the Qi Effect into everyday life is through fully understanding and embracing Heart Resonance. When we can quiet the Survival and Intellectual Minds and allow the Heart-resonant Intuitive Mind to guide us, our ability to activate Qi increases dramatically. Living a life guided by Heart Resonance is truly your path to freedom, love, and transformation.

Visit www.CommunityAwake.com if you would like to take the online Course on Heart Resonance and learn through audio and video support material.

Wuji Mountain Musings

This may be my most favorite chapter in this book. Maybe it's the chaotic and disjointed nature of it all. In that way, it represents life and the Qi Effect itself. It certainly represents my rebellious nature refusing to organize these Wuji Mountain musings into my earlier linear and coherent chapters. Wuji Mountain is an 8-acre sanctuary atop a forested mountain that I've been developing and where I've been living as a hermit, writing this book while building a boutique retreat facility as our non-profit CommunityAwake offering. Immersing in intentional isolation is a lot like fasting, it is a shift out of the comfort zone to allow body, mind, and spirit to ground, center, and return to clarity.

A longtime Taoist Qigong practitioner asked me recently, "How can there be a Wuji Mountain, a "mountain of nothingness"... I replied with a smile, "First, there was a mountain... and then, there was no mountain... and the monks sat and pondered this nothingness... and soon, there was again a mountain... Nothingness and Somethingness are but the same music playing on the well-tuned strings of our Heart..."

This may be considered the "Yin" part of the Qi Effect book, the gentle and feminine, non-linear aspect of the understanding I am here to share. Whereas the first part of this book is a bit more "Yang," a linear approach building step-by-step, Wuji Mountain Musings drop you into the energy we have built throughout this book and will allow you, if you are willing, to softly drift in that universe. In total, there are some 889 musings, and in this book we offer the first 108 - the rest are available in the actual Wuji Mountain Musings book itself. You are invited to explore these randomly as they follow no order and no logical flow... they serve only to nurture you and your Intuitive Mind. Some of you may enjoy flipping pages to see where you land while others of you may close your eyes, visualizing a number between 1 and 108 before opening your eyes to go to that number and seeing if you feel resonance with what you read. All are invited to select one or a few of the following offerings to use for group discussion with friends or during gatherings and classes. This is all from my Heart to yours...

Many people have collected the meaningful notes and bits that I had written them, and I have collected them here this chapter. I have added in many of the random, passing thoughts scribbled here or there in notebooks and on scrap pieces of paper. All of this touches into my Heart, and I am in deep gratitude to each person who has shared with me in this way knowingly or unknowingly. This comes as a reminder: we rarely know how we touch another person by what we say or write. When it comes from our Heart, it typically touches another Heart. We may never hear from that person again and we may have forgotten what was even said ... but the Third Field remains. Years later, someone may tell you how you positively affected their life by what you once shared with them. Maybe it even changed their life. This always reminds me of how important it is to stay as "Awake" and Heart-centered present as possible to the influence we have in this Dreaming we call life and personal interactions. The more we can speak from our Heart with the presence of Heart Resonance as our guide, the more of a chance we have to ignite that same Heart presence in another. This may be the most fundamental essence of the Qi Effect...

Enjoy this chapter. I do feel that reading the preceding chapters first will give you a contextual framework and lexicon for all that is presented before you here. It is a chaotic collection to be read in a random order and in an intuitively-guided fashion. I suggest you close your eyes and take a deep breath. Set an intention in the Qi field to receive exactly what serves your highest good and then open your eyes. Scroll down or open to one of the following pages of this introduction to the full Wuji Mountain Musings and give permission to your Survival and Intellectual Minds to take a break, trusting your Intuitive Mind to guide you to something that is meaningful for your spirit in the moment.

Breathe, Trust and have fun exploring...

1.

Integrating your life into your personal practice (Qigong, Tai Chi, Yoga, Meditation, whatever) is what this process of unfolding is all about.

Keeping anything "separate" from your practice is ego illusion and only reflects some fear response to why you don't trust enough to integrate it. You know in your intuitive Heartspace that ALL is energy... this maybe why you have had to "quit" your job or leave a relationship so that you can let go into this new life you are leading... It all will flow once you are Trusting the truth of this Dreaming... trusting that all is energy and it is for us, through our love and Heart-centeredness, to integrate our life's unfolding in a joyful and meaningful way... Ahh...

2.

Trusting in the harmonious alignment of both time and space is what we long to feel, to feel at peace with where we are in the moment. Only then will a love sensation emerge. This is when we begin accepting ourself, loving ourself, trusting ourself... This is beautiful. Accepting ourselves in this Dreaming we call life is such an amazing step... being able to say "Thank you for showing me the Edge of my Trust that I am Awake in my Dreaming..." This is when everything starts to shift... The "details" in the physical 3D world can never be "perfect" as that is not the nature of this dimension... BUT the essential energetic, the Source life-force is our perfect essence and that is what we are being asked to embrace. Doing this is what helps activate the Qi Field...

3.

Although frustrating, not fully sensing your Lower Dan Tian region in the belly is a blessed opportunity. Yes, medical challenges might identify certain blocks and stagnations there, so of course this would feel like a certain type of filter or fog that prevents you from feeling fully your energy at your core. This is when we are asked to activate the Qi Effect. When our body – which is like a channel or receptor – is operating in harmony, the Qi Effect expresses itself and we can seem to "feel" energy. Ample Qi energy is there already… it's simply for us to open to the sensing of it and thus, experience the healing benefits. This is our journey… and why we are attracted to Qigong practice so that we can continue to better prepare our body to be that healthy conduit channel for Qi Activation.

4.

The amount of time you practice is not as important as the quality of the time you spend in your practice… Trust… Yes, your sensitivity and intuition rises in proportion to transforming Fear into Intuition… Keep embracing this… Sensitivity is your power… and soon the emotions that rise up can be fully felt and then transformed… This is how we tap the power latent within them… Breathe deep…

5.

Trust that people who teach Qigong around the world reflect their own world views and are doing their best… many simply try to conform to what they read in books or heard from other teachers (who also read books or just listened to their own teachers.) There is a temptation to be "accepted" in any group of humans, and Qigong is no different than any other aspect of life… This drive to be accepted can many times come from the fear of NOT being accepted… and as we discussed – especially in Organ Cleansing Qigong - when Fear is UP, intuition is DOWN. When intuition (Heart wisdom, our Higher Self) is high, we see thing for the

Truth that they are: integrated, reflective, essential, unified, infinite… and perfect chaos… where all is possible. This is the essence of the term Wuji Hundun…

6.

Keep feeling your calm… your Practice is your teacher, yes… Your Trust will come with calm and calm will come with Trust… all this will keep flowing naturally from your practice… This is what people will keep seeing… Our personal practice is our mirror in the Dreaming…

7.

Your body will continue to soften as you transform your stress and sadness into Empathy… remember that is one of the core aspects of the Organ Cleansing Qigong principles - transforming emotion energy into useful fuel for our healing and empowerment. Empathy is a powerful and directive force, True Empathy allows you to "feel for" others but not "feel as" others… "Feeling" as is sympathy - just as in "sympathetic vibration," everything starts to vibe in the same way, creating a mess and not allowing anyone to see clearly. Empathy allows you to retain your core, your Awakened sense of self… this is truly how we heal… supporting and empowering others in the process…

8.

Instructor Certification is a "process" and it's not a "test-to-pass"… As with any "process," there are stages and a certain series of steps required to move through it. It's not only "quantitative" (i.e. # of hours) but "qualitative" (depth of awareness), and that takes a certain time and process to ascertain. The "qualitative" aspects are what makes Qigong Qigong after all… So much of what is involved in Qigong cannot be "quantified." Any high-level elder teacher I studied with "qualified" me to teach their form after years of training and observation, not by testing me on specific knowledge - most of which is in the realm of the Intellectual Mind anyway - but by observing me in how I shared a meal with them, how I taught their students, how I lived my life... how I expressed the theories and principles in who I was in this world...

9.

Yes, this journey of opening the pathway to our Heart can feel "painful" sometimes... Maybe that is simply our Identity, our survival drives, pushing back to secure it's position in the face of Fear... Breathing into that makes it all a bit easier, knowing that the process is natural and to be expected... and that allows us to "see" the flow from our Intuitive Mind, the Awakened Self... Trust this and keep shining as you do!

10.

You change and others will appear to change as well… and that is a treat to observe. It's like looking at a crystal from different angles... It's always the same crystal, but the appearance from a new perspective makes if feel "different." Enjoy every view as it all reflects you in some way!

11.

It is my honor to help and support those interested in opening their pathways to their Heart... it is my joy to support those on the journey to their sovereign authenticity... This is what helps us all remember we are on the same path... and yes, we are never alone. As my old teacher was fond of saying, "We are never alone, but we are 'all one'…"

12.

Sharing from your Heart and all that has been unfolding for you is rarely easy, even when we have been calling in all our mental, physical, emotional, and spiritual resources just to maintain some semblance of stability. This is the state of confronting our Edge. As painful as it is, it is a blessing. You are now standing at the mirror. What do you choose to see?

13.

Some things are not uncommon after deep spiritual or energetic training… it's as if we prepare ourselves for transformation and growth and until we are truly ready, the necessary life experiences don't come… The conclusion: You are ready for all this you are now experiencing.

14.

Maybe your humility is coming up as the path to your Heart is opening. You are tapping into your energy resources that will support you through any challenging phase. Instead of just "managing" the flow, you can use the energetic flux and chaos to transform, heal, and expand into your latent potential. This is potential that typically can't fully be accessed without being pushed to your Edge. The Edge shows us the path for rising the vibration to where it is required to be for the change to occur…

15.

Through all you experience in challenging times, it is important to do what it take to see our Anger transforming to Discernment… this is powerful and can only be done in Heart Resonance. This is how we "take action" and not "wallow." Your Heart resonant Intuitive Mind will naturally rise into your awareness and that is an excellent sign of transforming emotion, whether it is Anger into Discernment or Fear into Intuition.

16.

As for our Qigong, Yoga, or Tai Chi practice… releasing the need to be rigid in our self-expectation and embrace the joy of "taking small steps." Sometimes a "small" step is much more meaningful than a "big" step… Trust this… All steps lead you on your path and keep you moving forward… Gravitating toward your favorite and what for you are the most effective/joyful moves and asana is healthy and natural. I do it all the time. Challenging moves can be woven in as your build your foundation. Anyone who tells you otherwise may have ulterior motives. Trust… It is not about the particular movement, but rather the intention your carry in your Heart as you move…

17.

Work challenges (Edges) can be quite powerful – family ones too – these dig deep within us and bring up lots of emotion… but remember from the Organ Cleansing Qigong form that the Emotions carry power for us to access Qi/Prana. Activating that energy is key to our transformation.

18.

How beautiful that you have gained insights around your menstrual cycle… This is really fantastic. Remember the healing work that we did together? A lot of that was about releasing this feminine energy locked up inside you.

Freeing our Yin power brings clarity about our Truth and is a major step on our journey. For a big part of life, women are blessed with a monthly cycle that men are not. The feminine power of Yin is expressed in part to the physical – including water, the Earth and Moon, etc. – and this gives a unique power to women that men don't have. Instead, men can fall prey to use Yang force and "macho" compensation, which in the end, makes them much weaker than if they remember to express their Yin. Harmonizing our Yin (Feminine) and Yang (Masculine) is more that just cliché word use; it is key to our healing and transformation…

19.

How wonderful when physical flexibility and emotional flexibility can be seen as interwoven! Experiencing the inner strength and clarity that minimizes our trigger-reactions to others and keeps our judgement at bay is wonderful... Personal practice cultivates patience, a virtue as it has long been said...

20.

Feeling others empathetically rather than "sympathetically" is a big step. It allows us to stay sensitive and Heart-centered without getting into that "sympathetic vibration" with another and getting caught in – and affected by – their disharmony, their story.

21.

Your confidence will naturally rise as you come more into your self-love and core Heart presence.

22.

Understanding how to use your practice to bring calm and clarity to challenges in life is a blessing. This is one of the powerful aspects within the transformative nature of Qigong's conscious breathing and gentle movement practice. I love that in just minutes we can shift our emotions and bring ourself back into alignment and harmony. How committed are you to your practice?

23.

With time, we learn to secure that "Qi State" feeling that you get when you practice, and learn to call it up – access it – in the moment of your emotional trigger, what we call our Edge – the name for any challenge, pain, imbalance. When we first feel ourself going into that reaction mode after something happens to us or someone says something to us that upsets our mood, try to secure the feeling that you are cultivating in your practice. Maybe you have to walk out of the room and find a place to close your eyes. In that moment, breathe and with each breath, imagine that you are doing your Qigong practice. Don't actually do the movements in this exercise, simply feel the sensation of doing them. This can be very effective.

24.

Each time you have 20 minutes or so to actually do Qigong, Yoga, or Tai Chi exercises, remember that you are cultivating a memory, an energetic field memory, that you will be making available for the next time your Edge occurs. In this curious technique, you are making yourself aware that the "future" occurrence actually "exists" in the intention that you are setting in the present moment. This is powerful and transformative. Then, the next time the Edge takes place, you find that moment to close your eyes and you recall and access your practice's inner calm and harmony. Soon, with practice, the "two moments" (the Edge and your Practice) meld into one. You may be surprised what can happen with this awareness of "folding time" in a conscious, Awakened way.

25.

Embrace "shinjin ichinyo"… "Oneness of Body/Mind" is not so much of a "concept" as it is a "surrendering"… It about accepting the Truth that Body/Mind is a singularity, they are frequency bandwidths of the Infinite Consciousness that we are expressing in each moment of our existence. Qigong and Meditation are bridges into that "surrender" – a great word as it means to "give back"… as if we are giving back the idea/belief that Body and Mind are somehow separate and apart… and in its place, embracing our integrated Oneness…

26.

As we do our practice, feel how you are melting into sensation... Keep playing with the release of duality, where no longer are there "separate things" to even melt together... Surrender into seeing, feeling Body/Mind as a unified singularity... Breathe...

27.

Embrace the sensation of becoming more and more comfortable with your practice and feeling the Intellectual Mind's role less engaged... I feel this is part of why the ancients designed the moves in our practice... For one, they are optimized for accessing the Qi Effect – activating how life force engages with our physical body. Not only that, but the psychology of practicing a somewhat simple and repetitive movement is such that at the moment you no longer need to "think" about it, you've made a certain "leap" in perception. The neural pathways for the brain's motor function move into what some term "muscle memory," and our conscious Intellectual Mind is no longer required. It "tricks" this mind in a way and allows our Intuitive Mind to finally have a say in our flow without being pushed out by the controlling intellect. This is part of why we need to take time in our practice... It's actually quite wonderful to observe. Bringing the Intuitive Mind (we may call Higher Self but I prefer the former) into conscious awareness is the path to true freedom...

28.

It is not uncommon for health issues to appear more obvious after the focused practice you have been engaging in. First off, we are increasing our body-consciousness: our overall awareness and sensitivity is increasing as we wake up our Intuitive Mind. Secondly, as our Intuitive Mind becomes more engaged and Awake in our "normal" life, that awareness will "use" the body more as a "lexicon" to help communicate key aspects of what can support us in our spiritual transformation. This is one of the most fascinating aspects of Qigong and energy work in general. We tend to think that by doing these practices, everything in our body will instantly heal… but we forget that the body is a key communication device for showing us aspects of ourselves that impede our evolution - and many of those aspects have been lurking in us epigenetically throughout our ancestry. The good thing is that this is typically a transitionary stage in our personal development.

29.

When we face a physical/medical challenge with no true self awareness or understanding of the physical/emotional linkage, we are operating Asleep and primarily from the survival drives of our Survival Mind. We simply want the problem solved so we can get back to, well, survival. This is the endless, habitual loop of an empty life that most people mask through all the coping skills that modern life affords (drinking, drugs, mental chatter, entertainment, social media, etc.) Trusting our Heart Resonance will wake up deep wisdom within us, and is the only solution to finally transcend the loop.

30.

When we observe our illness and disease from our Awakened observer self – with the Intuitive Mind engaged – we see that challenge as an opportunity, a window into our spiritual life and evolution. It does not mean that we stop doing our best to take care of the situation and keep our body healthy… it means rather that we expand our perception to see the full dimension of what is taking place in our life. We begin to understand on the deepest level that our symptoms and challenges are "Edges" of our deepest Trust which are communicating something to us. We are being asked to listen and observe from the Intuitive Mind rather than the Survival Mind. Sometimes the ailment/challenge has a metaphoric quality to "what" it is – issues with vision can point to ways that we can "look" at our lives a different way for instance. Sometimes the ailment/challenge is being presented in a way that tests "how" we are reacting… and this can show us a lot on an emotional level. So whether it is "what" or "how" – and many times it is a combination of the two – it is this Awakened dimension to the Edge that we are being presented with that will lead us to true healing and spiritual development.

31.

Your practice will always continue to take on an energy of its own... that is why you feel so good when you practice. Being "here and now" is securing you into the Infinite Qi Field... it's only natural... You are sensing the "Qi Effect" I talk about... Sure, this Qi State euphoria can take you away from the world's challenges, but this is only the first stage... The key is to keep allowing this grounded sensation from your practice to influence the "normal world" of challenges and responsibility. Soon there will be no separation and your "practice" will blend into tasks at work and while with your family. You already feel this at times, allow it to continue...

32.

There is never a time in this body when we are "healed enough" to then go out and heal others... That is illusion, no matter what anyone says. Of course, one should never "do harm" to another by being in an unhealthy condition on a body, mind, or spirit level. Healing is an ongoing process in this Dreaming we call life. It is through being Awake enough to see ourself as an evolving, dynamic Qi Field that we can understand that "healing" others is truly an extension of seeing ourselves "healed." It is all part of our unfolding as Infinite Consciousness knowing itself through us... Trust this... and allow situations to arise where you share your healing influence/inspiration with others who can benefit...

33.

How wonderful when we can sense the influence of our own self love on the world around us... Seeing yourself as your Authentic and Sovereign Self, the Truth of who you are beyond body/mind, is a blessed insight. Embracing Infinite Consciousness, Source, expressing through us is such a key part of self love. Yes, all we experience relating to body/mind is under our responsibility in some way and is reflected in our choices we make everyday. All is a reflection of our awareness (consciously and subconsciously.) It's not that we necessarily "create" or "manifest" anything or any situation – but we are a BIG influencer... Embracing that responsibility is a gift... and a key to our unfolding and evolution... Stay with this flow...

34.

What can you be for others if you don't care and love for yourself first? How beautiful when we really see that. It's time to really and truly love yourself... We have been taught so much to care for others first, to not be "selfish"... and all that is good when you are caught in your Survival Mind... but when you are a sensitive soul and you naturally care for others, the directive shifts back to yourself. You find that putting yourself first, which can be a little challenging, is absolutely essential if you really care about others.

35.

Enjoy it... savor it... "Play" on this "plateau" we call joyful freedom... it is your playground... the place to be gentle with yourself and observe... Allow your Qigong practice to be just what it needs to be... just what flows. Allow it to be different from one day to the next... Allow it to have whatever quality emerges... Your practice is like taking care of a child, you keep enough boundaries to be safe, but keep enough flexibility to allow for growth potential to emerge... In this way, you can accept the child within you as well.

36.

Very responsible people need to remember to play… Enjoy your "playground" wherever it appears… usually it is just at the Edge of "self love," right?

37.

Observe the difference between your left hand and your right; this is how we build body awareness… This sensitivity assists us in our practice. It's wonderful when we can see how Qigong can help with our self "diagnosis"… this is part of the self awareness that naturally flows from building sensitivity to the inner listening of proprioception. "Diagnosis" isn't always about what is "wrong"… diagnosis can also tell you what is "right"… It is like a compass… it points you in a direction. Trust your Intuitive Mind and follow the trail you are being led on…

38.

Knowledge… If you are a responsible person with high integrity, it is clear you welcome knowledge. You want to do the best job you can when you teach, help, or just talk to others about a subject. Remember that knowledge from books, facts, and specific techniques can be helpful, but they can also create conflict since some people may disagree or have opposing views. We also need to be cautious not to let our Intellectual Mind Ego (i.e. Teacher Identity) pull us too far away from our Heart. The very best results supporting others - from friends and family to students - seem to always come from when you share from your Heart Resonance of the Intuitive Mind. Sharing your personal experience, your personal healing, your feelings, and your insights from your Heart will most often touch the Hearts of others. Once you establish that intention, then the "knowledge" aspects can emerge and they will be guided not by the intellect, but by your Heart.

39.

Learn to gently observe yourself in the process of assessing yourself...
This is how we learn and build up our sensitivity and intuition.

40.

The ancient way of looking at life was truly the Intuitive Mind at play...
and in this way, so many of the ancient mystics from seemingly disparate
cultures all seem to "see" things in curiously similar ways... A few cultural
overlays here and there can give you the illusion of separation between say
Taoism and Kabbalist mysticism, but at the core, the essence they arrived
at touches what I feel ARE the fundamental principles that underlie this
dimension where we live.... Keep feeling into the flow, beyond the details...

41.

Most times the "demons" we feel are the workings of our Survival Mind
and the Fear that drives that aspect of Mind. There is an aspect of each of
us that is truly Infinite and connected to the whole of the Universe. This
aspect of our Intuitive Mind is sometimes difficult to grasp, but we can get
glimpses and insights of it. It is difficult to grasp because our Intellectual
Mind and our Survival Mind (two other aspects of the full range of our
Mind potential) are vying for power and control. This is the human
condition. Our Intellectual Mind grasps for knowledge and facts to manage
Fear... while the Survival Mind is constantly on the watch for demons and
anything that could harm us. Watching this drama with a smile frees you
from it!

42.

Observe new concepts gently... without over-thinking, simply feeling
into them. Imagine if you could bring both of the drives that contribute

to Fear and Anger - the Intellectual Mind and the Survival Mind - and bring the energy behind these drives into your Heart. Allow that Fear to transform in your Heart Resonance and as it does, invite it to emerge as Intuition... waking up your Intuitive Mind. This Intuitive Mind – sometimes referred to as our Higher Self – is another frequency bandwith of the full range of Infinite Conscious that moves through us, that makes us who we are. Cultivating that Intuitive Mind from the power latent in Fear is a powerful part of the emotional alchemy in Organ Cleansing Qigong. Trust this. Meditate on this. It is what will free you. When Fear is transformed into Intuition, the energy (Qi) of that emotion is activated to empower us, to help wake up our potential. Keep trying this transformational exercise over and over and observe what occurs within you. Watch how the Survival Mind and the Intellectual Mind try their best to convince you (your Intuitive Mind) that they are right... This is the power of Fear... but knowing that we can tap into the power behind that Fear and transform it is a great gift and a life-changing process. Trust and put it to the test.

43.

In any chronic situation, we can pray that the "third time is a charm" as they say... What I mean here is that by seeing current trauma as part of an ongoing flow, we have the opportunity to look beyond "accident" or "illness" or anything simply "physical." Sure, there are absolute physical aspects to this flow, but I invite you to take this moment to consider looking deeper... Mostly because you don't want this "chronic" flow to continue... and also because you have an opportunity to facility real and lasting transformative healing...

44.

It's not always easy to look at life from a totally honest perspective as it can touch on some old wounds and emotional tender spots within us.

Trust in your Heart that this is a perfect time to transform your current situation and tap into the gift that is being presented to you...

45.

It's good to work in harmony with physicians as they are adept at the mechanics of tangible body parts and surgical repair... ..but YOU are adept at the subtle energy task of "flow" and "clearing" - especially as it relates to the energy of your own body... Trust you know your body better than any doctor... So continue with the docs for sure, but for the "deep" work - especially for chronic conditions, Qigong and energy healing is key...

46.

Try to shift your perspective that wants you to get Qi to "flow" through your body and organ systems... Instead, focus more on "seeing" your body and organ systems in perfect form and function, fully healed, and immersed in Qi... This is key to activating the Qi Effect... We are being asked to "embrace" the image of our body (and all organs, blood, nerves, connecting tissue, muscles, etc.) reflective of their inherent DNA-level "wisdom" which holds the design of your healthy "perfect" form and function. Coursing through you right now are stem cells that carry this perfect picture of you - this is science!

47.

Yes, life is a curious flow for sure... as the old Master I studied with back in the '70s used to say, "The Universe abhors a vacuum." In other words, as soon as a schedule or situation is cleared, many times, something rushes in to fill it.

48.

Yes, our whole life, every breath, is our "practice"... it never "ends" as it is always "beginning"... this is the beauty of it all... a rebirthing of sorts constantly as we engage with knowing Infinite Consciousness is knowing itself through our human experience, through our Intuitive Mind and then gently guiding our Intellectual Mind and our Survival Mind... Ahh... This is the nature of True Self, so yes, be happy with being with "your Self"...it is a magical journey of endless, loving discovery...

49.

"See" your Kidneys and other organ systems "immersed" in the Qi Field... nothing really needs to flow, Qi is already there, accessible to every atom in every molecule in every cell... Use your intention to activate the Qi Effect... to bridge Qi into your physical form... This is very effective....

50.

Forgiveness... 40+ years ago my old energy healing teacher would always say that "to forgive" really was to "give for" Turning the words around like that was like turning the energy around relating to the person you wished to "forgive"... "Give" up the old belief you held about the situation "for" a transformed, Awakened one... Transformed in the Heartspace of this Present Moment...... and many times, the "person" we need to "forgive" is ourselves...

51.

It's amazing how setting an intention can help ease your practice flow so that you can drop deeper into the "moving meditation" aspect of your Qigong. Observing the mind and how it sneaks in and judges is a curious thing... Trust... yes, building Trust within our spirit so that we can simply allow... and melt into that Wu Wei "effortless action" flow... After our Intellectual Mind did all its good work to help us learn the form... and our

Survival Mind did its work to keep us safe… both these aspects of Mind can ease up their hold and allow our Intuitive Mind to let us truly fly and expand into our essential self… Keep Trusting and flying…

52.

Trust that you are blessed to have the occasional frustrating student in your class or person in your world! 2,500 years ago, the Chinese moralist Confucius wrote, "What is a bad woman but a good woman's teacher." I don't like much of what Confucius believed in as it was extremely structured, but this message was a good one for me… Even the most challenging person offers us a great teaching opportunity to learn about ourselves! First, our sensitivity is our power… I don't believe we need to build a thicker shell to face the world. What I have learned is to go further into my sensitivity, not back away from it. This means to keep opening our Intuitive Mind… keep opening the pathway to our Heart. With this deeper sensitivity, we will be able to not only "feel" that frustrating person's Heart vibration, but connect with it/them in the process. Our ability to stay in Heart Resonance gives the other person the opportunity to do the same… and that's really why they have come into our Third Field. Within all the Ego-threatening aspects of the relationship that challenge the Survival Mind, there is a healing taking place… and the same goes for you since energy expresses itself in all directions. It's never a single person's contribution: two people make a relationship. That is where the true healing takes place. We are being asked to keep allowing our Shen Qi Heart energy field to engage. Each time we are triggered, I suggest you say "Thank you " to yourself and gently draw that feeling into your Heart… Yes, even during class or during a challenging encounter – Especially in the moment the trigger occurs if you can. You are clever, you can multi-task… this is one of the useful aspects of real sensitivity and empathy… Expand into that… There is a gift there for both you and the person you are sharing the Third Field with!

53.

Our parents are a major influence in both our Intellect Mind and Survival Mind conditioning. They typically didn't take the "spiritual path" that we have, so they are dominated by these two Mind influences. Their Intuitive Mind took a back seat and "spirituality" was primarily Fear-based or Intellect Mind at work. It's an oversimplified explanation, but useful. Allow your parents and their ways to be a supportive aspect of your growth... Wrap gratitude around your ability to "See/Feel" this perspective from your Intuitive Mind viewpoint... It's very much worth the journey and exploration...

54.

Guided Meditations are very empowering, especially for those who can tap into the visuals and for those that are not always comfortable sitting in "quiet." I've had decades of training in temples and with monks and know the effectiveness of consuming the "monkey mind" with a mantra or chant.... Guided Meditation serves that end as well.

55.

As my first elder teacher used to remind me, "You teach best what you need to learn most."

56.

Sometimes what we think are "little steps" are really "quantum leaps." You may not see this at first. Why? We tend not to be grounded in our self-worth and are usually self-judgmental. What is more "grounding" than embracing the infinite space of our Heart? What builds confidence and a greater sense of our True Nature than aligning with Heart-centered intention? Yes, being gentle with yourself is the first step. By allowing that to become natural and consistent, people who trigger us become so much easier to "see" for who they are... and what they awaken in us...

57.

Relationships are such beautiful places to observe our Edges... and when we can feel our Heart Resonance within, we are allowing more space to express our Truth with others. Curious how we can forget this at times. It is natural to forget, and can have many deep rooted reasons from the past. But so what? The details aren't quite as important as embracing your sovereign nature in this moment, loving yourself, seeing that you are beautiful and authentic just as you are – as an expression of Infinite Consciousness knowing itself through you. That may sound a bit heady and out-there, but you know what this means. Getting clear that we are Awake in this amazing Dreaming, we have all the energy required for our evolution, all the Qi access required for our transformation... when we truly engage in coming from Heart space. It's wonderful when we can embrace that, even for a moment, and our Intuitive Mind shines and the causal roots of our challenges may appear. With Heart-centeredness, they can be seen for what they are: limited perceptions from an conditioned Survival Mind. Waking up to this is a critical part of our development and evolution, and allows relationships to blossom in new and beautiful ways.

58.

Ahhh, one step forward, two back... so what? Who's counting? The Survival Mind? She's what got you into trouble in the past, so why listen to her any longer? Our Intuitive Mind operates on Heart Resonance, and she doesn't even know how to count – and she's terrible with direction and time! She only knows one thing, Love and presence in this moment. These steps all become part of a beautiful dance... your dance, your transformation asking you to enjoy the journey without judgement..

59.

Moving into Autumn and cooler weather asks us to be gentle with our bodies... Flow with it... It's the shamanic Taoist way to appreciate how to

shift with the seasons… Go at the pace of your Heart… she knows. This is
a big piece of our self-confidence… For relationships that are challenging
and even abusive, it simply means that we have allowed Fear or Anger to
shield our Heart. Trust that confidence simple means "with trust" (from
the Latin root)…and confidence can really only come from being Heart
centered… That is your power… move at the pace of your Heart… keep
listening, you'll know…

60.

When emotions arise and seem to overwhelm us, it's at that instance
that they need to be felt with a conscious breath, named, and then brought
into Heart space… This is Qigong's Emotion Alchemy… Yes, embracing
Hundun chaos puts it all into harmonious alignment… knowing that this
is the nature of this 3D world… and trusting that within that chaos is
Infinite Consciousness and a curiously perfect order… Chaos itself is the
force behind creation itself, for new beginnings… It is for us to stay Awake
to this and remember our True nature… Infinite Consciousness knowing
itself through our human experience. Breathe into that… it changes
everything and helps us stay Awake in this Dreaming... True confidence
emerges from this grounded Heart Resonance.

61.

Stay with your personal practice… however you feel comfortable with
the flow… Allow Qigong or Tai Chi or Yoga to be your safe space for
transformation… Allow that practice time to embrace and consume all
of you and allow it all to move from Intellectual Mind to Intuitive Mind.
Through your practice, the Shen Qi Field of spirit will become more and
more evident and tangible. The fact is, it's there now, patiently waiting for
your embrace and acceptance…

62.

The most wonderful miracles are simple, barely perceptible... This is true Wu Wei - "No Action"... the infinite embodied in every subatomic particle... every grain of sand... the subtle shifts in the way we move or breathe... These are the miracles I embrace... Trust this more and more, and as you do, your life path will continue to reveal itself as will the embrace of your True Nature, that Authentic Self that brings us ease and confidence... It is such a curious journey this life... and to see ourselves in the context of Infinite Consciousness knowing itself through us, through our human experience, helps put it all into a sweet context... so that a simple movement combined with breath becomes everything, and at once, nothing... This is what frees us... This is what allows us to see that we are already fully healed.

63.

It is your Heart connection that will continue to help you access your Intuitive Mind... As our Survival Mind and Intellectual Mind come into peace, the bandwidth opens to our Intuitive Mind... This is where intuition lies... it's always there, it's just a matter of accessing it. Trust... the pathway is through your Heart Resonance... Your consistent practice will reveal this to you in every way.

64.

We are all one... This is the Judeo-Christian (and Muslim as well) principle of seeing others as Jesus reminded us, as brothers and sisters, as the same children of God. This brings great peace as we begin to trust that we are all on this path of evolution and unfolding together. Some are more Awake than others... and the fact is, the majority of people are Asleep... This is not a judgement, but an observation. They are trapped in the cage of their Survival Mind and/or their Intellectual Mind conditioning, and this burden dictates a certain set of responses and behaviors. As Buddha also reminds us, when we can release ourselves from the desire bred from that conditioning, each of us can attain the oneness of nirvana.

65.

We explore what we refer to as the Edge… our challenges of Trust. Although not the most fun part of our journey, the Edges are in fact where we evolve, where we develop Trust, where we learn to truly engage our Heart and activate the Shen Qi Field Effect. When an Edge is met – either gently observed or overtly presented to us (like a challenging financial situation or health condition) it is an opportunity to grow. I like to take three steps: 1) Say thank you and express gratitude for the ability to see the situation as an Edge, the boundary of my Trust; 2) I name the emotion that comes up – this helps to make it objectified and tangible and prepare for the next step; 3) Draw that emotion you've named into your Heart, into that powerful presence of your Intuitive Mind. This step can be supported with breathing and Qigong to great benefit. When in Heart space, allow that Survival Level emotion to be seen as a bridge, a vehicle, of the fuel required for your transformation. Recall what Awakened State that emotion takes in Heart space (Fear/Intuition; Anger/Discernment; Grief/Empathy; Worry/Clarity) and then feel into that Awakened State of the emotion, utilizing the Qi Effect fuel that came with it. Allow your Heart to embrace the feeling… to transform whatever comes up in the process… Stay present and expansive. This is a powerful exercise, and part of the Organ Cleansing Qigong practice.

66.

Allowing Hundun to express itself is a wonderful joy. Being at peace with chaos is such a great sign of our practice evolving. Trusting the Perfection woven into the chaos is how we learn to fully tap into and access the Qi Effect. This means that on a mental and physical level, we can fully allow the Qi Field to be activated. We move beyond the "normal" activation (that which keeps everyone alive – even if just on a survival level) and begin to experience higher and higher percentages of the Qi Effect in our lives. This activates healing on a mind, body and spirit level as it activates our Intuitive Mind.

67.

Our personal practice touches many aspects of our life and it is a blessing to observe the benefits that come with dedicated and sincere practice. The challenge is that most of us are immersed in Survival and Intellectual Mind activity and view our practice through that lens. The more we can embrace Heart-centered practice, the more we are gently guided into the Intuitive Mind space. From that intuitive place, we realize we have so many tools that actual support our survival and intellect! That is the curious paradox of it all. It is seductive to allow the Survival and Intellectual Minds to take over, but they are typically driven by Fear and Anxiety. Only the Intuitive Mind transcends Fear as it emerges from Heart Resonance. Keep allowing your Shen Qi – that Heart-centered vibration of spirit – to guide you. Trust and your confidence will grow…

68.

It is natural to be frustrated by the "vision" we have for our life, especially when things actually look very different than your "vision" in the present moment… Yes, on one level, they can appear in conflict… On another level, the two are dancing together on the mirror of your life choices… Your Survival Mind sees the two "visions" (where you would like to be and where you are now) as opposites and in conflict, and resolves to keep you where you are. Even your Intellectual Mind is agreeing with that, judging and adding the logic that maybe you just should resolve the issue by waiting for more data! Ahhh… All this wakes up your Intuitive Mind – that part of your Mind that hasn't been given a chance to share in the discussion because she has been bullied by the other two very assertive aspects of Survival and Intellectual Mind. So much for teamwork! So, now it is time to recognize this, find some quiet, and kindly ask your Survival Mind and Intellectual Mind to relax and be quiet so that your Intuitive Mind can have her say. This sounds like a curious process, but Trust me, it is very effective. Keep reminding your Survival Mind that you very much appreciate her great contribution to keeping you fed and housed… and keep reminding your Intellectual Mind that her logic has been very sound and helpful... Let "them" know that in this exercise, you need them to know they have very little to contribute because they've done their jobs so well... and that this time is for your Intuitive Mind to have her chance to share in how to make your "vision" Heart-centered and valid.

69.

Some things take a few attempts... but the moment will come when – maybe with your eyes closed and a warm cup of tea in your belly – your Intuitive Mind will start speaking out. You'll know her because she has no concerns with basic survival needs... nor does she rely on intellect or logic. She is your Higher Self coming directly from your Heart Resonance. Allow the spirit space that the ancients called Shen Qi to simply express without judgement or fear... and if those two come up, simply say "thank you" and return to your centered Heart...

70.

The more you allow your Intuitive Mind to share, the more you will begin to receive what we'll call "downloads" about solutions and strategies for the changes necessary to your life for your personal evolution. Trust this. When these so called "solutions" come from the Survival Mind or Intellectual Mind, they are wrought with conditioning limits, fear, and logic. Breathe into this... and return to trusting your Heart.

71.

Get to know your inner voices so that you can start to identify where your thoughts are coming from. This is very important... Each Mind bandwidth has its role to allow us to live in this world... but only the Intuitive Mind is of the Heart frequency that supports our Transformation.

72.

It is easy to get consumed by the Intellectual Mind… but it is also natural to ask and inquire… Teachers say kids can't read without knowing the whole alphabet. Sure, we need to know what each letter sounds like so that we can pronounce a word… but I know many children who can read and still don't know all the letters… It's not until a new word appears with a new letter in it that they joyfully expand their understanding… This is a nonlinear approach to discovery. Qigong really doesn't have an underlying linear structure and it's gift is that it is a flowing nonlinear path of exploration providing amazing benefits. That's what baffles the linear Intellectual Mind. Mapping linearity onto non-linearity is exactly why the modern medical world gets so frustrated with Qigong!

73.

Early in our practice, we begin to embrace that our "mind" influences Qi life force energy. This begins to describe the power of intention. I personally do not believe that Qi actually "moves" anywhere. As I say many times in my workshops, we are immersed in an Infinite Field of Qi energy. Our task in Qigong is to activate the Qi Effect – activate the way Qi interacts with our body for healing and rejuvenation. Movement, positive intention, and intentional breathing all contribute to this Qi Effect. Qi can appear to flow, but only to the untrained perspective.

74.

Tai Chi is typically a competitive form… People practice it in competitions and there are judges judging contestants for their precision. Though this aspect has very little to do with Qigong, Tai Chi is derived from it. Tai Chi Chuan was more of a martial art for self defense. This aspect also has very little to do with Qigong, but there is a soft and deep way to practice Tai Chi that transcends the martial influences and is very empowering. There, you can see how it merges with Qigong's "moving meditation" and evolved out of the same ancient healing and spiritual roots.

75.

Qigong is taught by many people who gain much from teaching precision and technique. It feeds the Intellectual Mind – and even the Fear-aspects of the Survival Mind. That's typically why so many people cling to these types of teachings. Typically they don't go very far in their development, other than becoming very precise. This rigidity rarely feeds the Heart. If you wish to pursue a path of precision, Intellect and Fear, then that is a personal choice… not better or worse than any other. My path is one of Transformation… moving out of the mess and confusion of the Survival/Intellectual cages that we have been trapped in. It's not to say that this path is for everyone. You will find many who wish to debate this and will spend a lot of time trying to convince me that their precision, principles, technique, and logic is correct and right. I have no issue with that and believe everyone should follow what they believe. The sad thing is that it is always what we believe that defines our world.

76.

The question then comes to, Is your world all you wish it to be? Is your body as healthy as you would like it to be? Are you as Heart-centered as you would like to be? Are your emotions as harmonious as your Joy requires? Ask these and then listen with your Heart resonance…If the answer to these types of questions are ever in the negative, then it's time to re-evaluate what you believe to be true…

77.

To say that everything is exactly the way it 'should be' is a very charged statement… It begs the question, "According to who?" You can say instead,

"Everything is exactly the way it is."… Now that has everything to do with being in the present and embracing what is so. That is a very Heart-centered statement that allows one to accept the moment at hand and draw up all your focus to begin your Transformation, which always requires the pathways to the Heart to be clear and open. It is only in the Heart where we transform Survival-based emotions into Awakened, Intuitive emotions.

78.

Everything is energy at the most fundamental level (in science we may say at the subatomic level). Qigong simply means the practice (Gong) of being in alignment with energy (Qi). When we are in alignment with energy, everything we do involves refining how we activate our relationship with Qi. To the beginner Mind, our thoughts "guide" Qi… with experience, we become in full alignment with Qi. This is the difference I discuss between being a "Container" and being a "Conduit."

79.

I ask you to meditate on your myriad ideas and questions, and revisit them gently as all are very well thought out from your very adept Intellectual Mind. I must say, it is this very Mind that gets us all into the most trouble… I will take time to answer your specific questions about the Wuji Hundun moves at a later time when I can fully respond. I will share that Master Duan always said to simply breathe naturally during the moves – with no specificity. I suggest, as a guide, to exhale with out and down movements, and inhale during in and up movements… It's a good starting place…. I also remind that, in accordance with what I shared before about Qi being infinitely present, that there is no actual Qi Emission – even though the majority of the Qigong world would like to believe this. Refer back to my explanation of Qi Effect Activation.

80.

I have lived in China for many years and studied with many, many Masters. Nearly every one of them contradicted each other – from Qigong to Tai Chi and Feng Shui to Tui Na. This is why there are SO many different factions and systems. This only proves to me that any specificity is inherently deviant from the essential principle. Lao Tzu is attributed as to saying that the Tao you can describe is not the Tao. The genius of the ancient Taoist wizards was to help people get introduced to concepts that were non-linear and open up that Intuitive part of us. Many who didn't comprehend this tried very hard to systematize Taoist concepts while still call themselves Taoists. Taoism became a religion and a science... and actually, it is neither. If we fall prey to this, we too will have to accept either the religious or scientific diversions of Taoism. By doing so, we will miss the gift that dances at the core of these concepts. Why did Lao Tzu ride off on his ox after writing the Tao Te Ching (as the story goes)... Symbolically it represents that after these concepts are even expressed, you must turn your back on them and leave... To stay and elucidate or to try and refine them would only attempt to impose linearity on the non-linear.

81.

Life is a Dreaming wide awake... and our sleeping dreams are clear and open windows to our subconscious. Listen to them and their metaphoric symbology... Our brilliant subconscious taps into our Survival and Intuitive Minds. Embracing the visions with an open Heart will always provide us with insight... and it always speaks to our personal transformation and growth... Ahhh...

82.

Nature is a fabulous mirror to remind us, just as our body is also a mirror... a mirror of our flow, our choices, providing us with insights and hints about our life journey. You will polish the mirror because of the dedication you have for your personal development: your path of self-discovery through meditation and practice.

83.

The Ego plays out through the Survival Mind, pushing us to want "more" as you say… It can't perceive itself unless it compares in duality and scarcity. It looks outward and defines itself through the world, always needing, grasping… and the Intellectual Mind defines the Ego as well, through judging and comparison. It is only when we can allow the Intuitive Mind to express itself that we can depart from the Ego-separation and merge with the world from a Heart-centered life. This is what Qigong helps to bring us to… opening the pathways to the Heart, inviting the Wei Qi Field to be fed by the Heart's Shen Qi Field… and with the Heart path clear, emotions can enter and be transformed… we can stay Awake in this amazing Dreaming we call Reality… It is why you love your Qigong time with your "tribe" during group practice…

84.

Qi is activated when you draw your Lao Gong up the inside of your leg along the Spleen Meridian… and yes, you are also activating Spleen Qi when you do the Stomach Cleansing and Strengthening move as your Lao Gong is again activating Spleen Qi since the Stomach and Spleen are complementary Yang/Yin organ systems… yet the other Yin organs (Liver & Kidney) and their complementary Yang partners will also be benefitting. Remember, it's not always about the "precise proximity" of your Lao Gong points when it comes to clearing and strengthening through Qi Activation… This is where our Yi comes in, where our ability to Activate Qi through intention becomes an effective tool and the specificities of having to place your hand in a specific spot for a specific length of time become less and less important… Trust this…

85.

Your self observation through the Heart Resonance lens will alway lead you to see yourself in a whole new way as a Conduit, and with that comes the freedom and healing you've been seeking. The power of our Intention is amazing, and learning to Activate Qi this way truly cuts through a lot technical and Intellectual conditioning barriers that we seem to create for ourself when we impose unnecessary finite limits on Qi.

86.

Part of your Self Love Program is about moving out of the "constant rush and feeling obligated" mode of life… and starting to following the rhythm of your Heart.

87.

Breathing… yes… I would say that breathing – and our consciousness around breathing is ALWAYS important… but it does change and evolve as we do. Master Duan's approach was to resist telling people what to do and rather push them to self discovery. That was his true Taoist side, and the one we all seek to cultivate. Learning the dimensions of breath is the journey… enjoy discovering this. When breath becomes cellular (actually subatomic), we have awakened our awareness to the essence of Qi Activation.

88.

The Tao is such that when we wake up to who we truly are, we find ourselves in the most interesting situations... It's no longer ego-survival driving us separate and against the world, we enter an Intuitive Mind Qi space where we ARE the world...

89.

Many times in life we get involved in something that reminds us that it's truly the "journey" and not the "destination." Keep this in your

Heart Mind as you release this dove of your intention into the sky... it will land where it is best received and you have to trust this. Your spirit of 'truthful diplomacy' (sometimes that seems like an oxymoron) is evident and our joint intention is that that this congealing of so many important, empowering and timely concepts will nudge along the glaciers and tanks. Trust everything is in harmony in this Dreaming we call life... Even in apparent conflict or stagnation there is still harmony... every energetic structure is in resonance where they fit in the moment... and yes, karma has much to do with this, whatever that is...

90.

You are supported in more ways than you can imagine... but keep imagining regardless!!!

91.

Activation and Clearing are essentially synonymous in the context of energy healing... Activation is the process of using Yi intention and specific field manipulation (instigated as hand positions, body posture, and breathing) to enhance and rarify the relationship between Qi AND aspects of the physical body. These "aspects" include cell activity, metabolic processes, organ function, respiration, flow dynamics, endocrine interactivity, genetic communication, molecular biochemistry, and even atomic/subatomic energetics. "Clearing" in this context is the transformation, moving, and redistribution of all that occurs to deter the smooth and efficient function of the above "aspects of the physical body." Yes, there are "blocks and stagnation" that need to be "cleared" - but I recommend that we move away from the disempowering belief that it is Qi that is blocked. Qi doesn't "flow" so it can't be "blocked." Qi isn't constrained by the physics of 3D materiality in this dimension... if it were, it wouldn't be Qi and it could be quantified... which no one has been able to do. We can certainly see the effect of Qi - this is nearly commonplace. We see obvious and quantifiable shifts in "aspects of the physical body." You see how I am emphasizing that phrase? It is because what we are "Clearing" are the aspects of the physical functionality that "Activating" the Qi Effect does so superbly...

92.

Grounding... Inhaling through the nostrils ensures the in-breath is warmed and hydrated (and somewhat cleansed by the fine hairs in the nostrils.) Exhaling through the nostrils AND mouth ensures complete expelling of as must CO_2 as possible. Try it out by exhaling with only the nostrils, and then open your mouth and blow out... if any air comes out, then there should be a benefit of opening the mouth on exhales for various breathing exercises.

93.

When circling your hands at the Lower Dantian region, let the speed fit with your breath... Actually, it is good to observe the speed as it sometimes indicates your state of mind like a barometer... Adjust in whatever way can assist you with the intention of entering a harmonious state of presence. This is why THIS is the first move of Organ Cleansing Qigong...

94.

Videos are a fixed and linear instruction, which can be quite constricting compared to live classes that help us understand the inherent flexibility related to many aspects of Qigong forms - including direction, speed, and handedness... Start with either right or left hand - and as I suggest, mix it up regularly to help you stay present...

95.

When stepping out to the side, it is best to step out with the "empty" leg. This means anchoring and sinking into the grounding, weight-bearing leg, and then stepping out with the opposite one that has minimal weight-bearing responsibility at that point.

96.

It is useful and necessary to pause in between moves to help digest and integrate what is taking place… but when you are playing Qigong with those who know the form (or if you are doing it on your own) it is a joy to move in a contiguous way where one move blends smoothly and elegantly into the other like a dance… Qigong is a mystical dance after all…

97.

In the compression phase of "Embracing Yin & Yang" in the Organ Cleansing Qigong form, I teach it in a way to keep people upright at first so they stay conscious of their core and don't just "lean over." Compress deep, drawing up the perineum and tightening your abs so that your lower dan tian region is activated. Once people are conscious of this intent, then there can be flexibility in the move…

98.

With Lung Cleansing and Heart Cleansing moves, longer breaths are quite acceptable if you can engage that naturally. Observe and see what will benefit you most… Elders with shorter breaths benefit and welcome breaking the moves into two shorter breaths.

99.

The breathing in the Stomach Cleansing move is quite similar to the Liver Cleansing breath… they both follow the same principle… Typically, downward/outward movements go with exhales while upward/inward movements go with inhales…

100.

In the Intestine Clearing move, I prefer leading with the Pinky and palm down/outward… It feels better and more effective.

101.

For the Gall Bladder/Nervous System Cleansing move, I bring my hands back to the energetic field of the Lower Dan Tian before moving into the Balancing/Harmonizing move. For that move, it is most effective for the hands to go out to the side, Lao Gong points facing down and then sinking into the Earth. I prefer not to say "gather Qi" but rather, "connect and integrate with the Earth Qi field"… it is much more empowering and less scarcity-oriented. To "gather" means that you "need something" when in fact we are immersed in an infinite Qi field… Keeping your feet wide here is fine… just observe students and be sure no one has knee issues that can be better addressed by bringing the feet closer together…

102.

In the Organ Cleansing form, we move through Meridian Cleansing near the beginning and again near the end. You can start Meridian Cleansing either on the right side or the left side. Notice how for the closing move, I usually switch the starting hand to help break the pattern of always "starting on the right." The key: Stay present and aware and try your best not to fall into unconscious patterns!

103.

The Closing Movement is a critical part of the Organ Cleansing form, and to me is the most necessary for integration and staying centered in a place of grounding and gratitude.

104.

Embracing the limiting notion of "Qi flow" takes trusting our Intuitive Mind. The more we can wake up to our Heart Mind wisdom, the less the effort of the Intellectual Mind is needed and we seem to have much more energy to access true wisdom. We don't need to "wake up," "build" or "flow" Qi at the Meridian level. Qi is infinite and ever-present, it simply needs to be activated. When it is, we can sense this activation around our body and it appears to "flow." We are being asked to wake up to our true energetic identity, wake up to the latent abilities of a Heart-centered Intuitive Mind in order to see this about Qi... This is the ONLY Identity worth nurturing... With that clarity, you can play with ANY identity you wish because none of them will ever be able to attach to you due to the energetic Teflon nature of the Heart... Ahhh...

105.

It is a blessing when your practice takes on a life and timing of its own... To me, that is always best. I get nervous when people get too regimented... Keep letting if flow. As we trust our Intuitive Mind more and more, we realize that the Heart is a phenomenal "translator." The Heart can take concepts or even apparent conflicting rules, and translate them into essence. This is big. Those caught in their Intellectual Mind space will piss and moan and spit blood at times, but my Heart allows me to smile and understand...

106.

From chaos emerges change... as a wonderful Nobel Laureate once told me after he received his award, "All biologically evolving systems must reach a point of maximum perturbation (i.e. chaos/hundun) before reaching their next higher level of order."

107.

Our karma is bound to, amongst other things, our ability to disentangle the bonds of epigenetic entrainment... So is the path of the soul in this dimension. We are asked to attend to what we CAN do... and in the process, stay true to our path.

108.

Yes, Qigong practice - including meditation, Tai Chi, and Yoga - is key to helping us "see" this world in a clear way. Life can be quite complex for all of us, we each are delivered a unique experience set called life that is tailored to us based on our choices and karma... it's what we do in that flow that makes us who we are...

———————

...and so goes the journey... an infinite and juicy one that asks us to question gently without seeking answers and adventuring without being obsessed with the final destination, as every point along the way is a destination in and of itself... Breathe deep... Love and Peace...

La Fine

Endorsements

"A magical mystery tour. Such an amazing piece of work. Using insights into science and ancient healing traditions gained over a lifetime of study, practice, and teaching, Francesco guides us in an exploration of the energetic nature of our reality through sensitivity training in life-force energy for health, healing, and self-care."
—Tom Rogers, President of the Qigong Institute, author of <u>An Introduction to QigongHealth Care</u>

"Francesco Garripoli has dared going beyond the traditional assumption that Qi originates and operates only within the boundaries of the space/time dimension we know so well. He bravely transcends this reductionistic concept and suggests there is an all-encompassing oneness that our soul knows, has no boundaries, and unimagined potential. Francesco invites us to join him in exploring the limitless dimensions of our human potential. Bravo Francesco!"
— Len Saputo, MD. Author, healer. www.DoctorSaputo.com

About the Author:

With over 40 years of studying, researching, and practicing the healing arts after his initial pre-med university training, Francesco Garri Garripoli is an author, musician, visionary, wellness advocate, Certified Senior Qigong Teacher and Chairman Emeritus of the National Qigong Association (NQA) and the current Chairman of the Qigong Institute. He produced the PBS-TV documentary, "Qigong: Ancient Chinese Healing for the 21st Century" and founded the nonprofit CommunityAwake organization.